The Social Dream-Drawing Workshop

The Social Dream-Drawing Workshop is a pioneering, practical guide for professionals who work with people going through major life transitions, such as career change, relocation or bereavement. These transitions can evoke enormous feelings of uncertainty and are times of vivid dreaming.

Social Dream-Drawing is a highly effective method of group work that mobilizes the dream's enormous capacity to help us adapt to life, whatever challenges it throws at us. This user-friendly book explains the underlying key concepts and basic steps of the Social Dream-Drawing method, from sharing dream drawings in a group environment to running digital sessions. It shows how these expressive drawings can bring an otherwise internal experience out into the open and serve as lifelong mementos of key times in our lives.

Including drawings and testimonials from workshop participants and guidance on creating a safe and supportive environment, *The Social Dream-Drawing Workshop* will appeal to therapists and counsellors as well as social workers, coaches and anyone interested in exploring this fascinating practice.

Dr. Rose Redding Mersky has been an organizational development consultant, supervisor and coach for over 30 years. She lives in Germany.

'What a delightful and erudite journey we are taken on as we engage with this text about dreams and drawings of dreams. Dr. Mersky elucidates the process and logistical aspects of Social Dream-Drawing through personal experience with and research about this method - sharing verbatim comments and drawings of the dreamers. She shows how SDD can create a safe containing space for participants to access below the surface material for individual and collective sense-making. She shares her expertise and wisdom about accessing our vulnerability and strength as facilitators using this method in various contexts, even online. Indeed, an urgent read if you want to start working with or even expand your work with dreams!'

Michelle S. May, *Professor in the Department of Industrial and Organisational Psychology, University of South Africa and Registered Clinical Psychologist at the Health Professions Council of South Africa*

'A unique book about one of the most accessible and incredibly effective methods for reaching deep and meaningful insights and achieving change in both personal and professional areas of life. Dream-Drawing offers a royal road to a deeper understanding of individual and group requests, identification of hidden limitations, and the discovery of the resources necessary to meet objectives. This method will not only help psychology students to master their future profession, but give them an important practical tool for future use. It is especially helpful in difficult and uncertain situations when the consultant senses vulnerability and helplessness. By receiving support from the clients' unconscious in the form of drawings of their dreams and associations to them, the consultant acquires the necessary resources and understanding of both the organizational request and the ways to resolve it'.

Professor Rossokhin Andrey Vladimirovich, *Department of Psychoanalysis and Business Consulting, HSE University, Moscow*

'With expertise that ranges from psychoanalysis to dreams to drawing and visual representation, Rose Redding Mersky has brought her substantial skills to bear on a fascinating and important topic. Combining erudite scholarship with practical explanation, she has produced a wonderful volume that tells you everything you need to know about Social Dream-Drawing. The book is filled with fascinating examples and is illustrated by some very poignant drawings. It is a joy to read - I cannot recommend it too highly'.

Professor Mark Stein, *Chair in Leadership and Management, University of Leicester, UK*

'What a truly delightful and authoritative book on an approach to drawing your dreams as an investigative tool which, as the drawing evolves, brings the dream material out into the open. It furthermore provides a creative means for visually sharing and working with your dreams in a social setting. SDD is not only a brilliant approach but the book clearly explains step by step how to adopt this approach as part of your personal, group and even virtual dream working experience. Very highly recommended'.

Bob Hoss, *Past President of the International Association for the Study of Dreams and Director of the DreamScience Foundation, USA*

'In this very accessible manual, Rose Mersky articulately yet simply captures the mystery and value of working with dream-drawings with groups of people going through major life transitions. The careful detail and sensitive elucidation in this step-by-step guide provides very helpful instructions for consultants interested in utilising this intriguing application of social dreaming – while also attending to the contribution of unconscious group dynamics. This is a fascinating account which includes many examples of social dream-drawings and the ways in which they assisted the participants to explore their concerns and apply their learning'.

Allan Shafer MA (Clinical Psychology) D Litt et Phil, *Socioanalyst & Psychoanalytic Psychotherapist, former President, Group Relations Australia*

'Dream drawing can enlighten your personal situation in many new and exciting ways, as it did for me in a workshop led by Rose, helping me to change my perspectives on our family business and to initiate processes that built a whole new level of trust within both our business and family'.

Christiane Wenckheim, *Chairman, Ottakringer Getränke AG, Austria*

The Social Dream-Drawing Workshop

A Handbook for Professionals

Rose Redding Mersky

Routledge
Taylor & Francis Group

LONDON AND NEW YORK

Cover image: Dream-drawing by Netherlands' participant Karien

First published 2023
by Routledge
4 Park Square, Milton Park, Abingdon, Oxon OX14 4RN

and by Routledge
605 Third Avenue, New York, NY 10158

Routledge is an imprint of the Taylor & Francis Group, an informa business

British Library Cataloguing-in-Publication Data
A catalogue record for this book is available from the British Library

Library of Congress Cataloging-in-Publication Data
Names: Mersky, Rose Redding, author.
Title: The social dream-drawing workshop : a handbook for professionals /
    Rose Redding Mersky.
Description: Abingdon, Oxon ; New York, NY : Routledge, 2023. | Includes
    bibliographical references and index.
Identifiers: LCCN 2022009967 (print) | LCCN 2022009968 (ebook) |
    ISBN 9780367225629 (paperback) | ISBN 9780367225605 (hardback) |
    ISBN 9780429275647 (ebook)
Subjects: LCSH: Dreams--Therapeutic use. | Group therapy. | Adjustment
    (Psychology)
Classification: LCC RC489.D74 M47 2023 (print) | LCC RC489.D74
    (ebook) | DDC 616.89/165--dc23/eng/20220629
LC record available at https://lccn.loc.gov/2022009967
LC ebook record available at https://lccn.loc.gov/2022009968

ISBN: 978-0-367-22560-5 (hbk)
ISBN: 978-0-367-22562-9 (pbk)
ISBN: 978-0-429-27564-7 (ebk)

DOI: 10.4324/9780429275647

Typeset in Times New Roman
by KnowledgeWorks Global Ltd.

To my dear husband and colleague,
Burkard Sievers

Contents

Acknowledgements

First, to Jasmine, who provided the original inspiration for this method by her marvellous dream drawings of myself and my client. Second, to my late colleague, Karien van Lohuizen, who hosted the very first Social Dream-Drawing workshops in her office in Haarlem. And to my two intrepid doctoral supervisors, Anne-Marie Cummins and Lita Crociani-Windland. Without them, there would be no book. And to the many colleagues who have supported me in this endeavour over all these years: Martina Jochem, Louisa Brunner, Verena Mell, Ullrich Beumer, Eduardo Acuna, Michelle May, Nigel Williams, Francesca Cardona, Simon Tucker, Pauline van Noort, Kalina Stemanova, Katya Shapovalova and Georges De Mullewie. And definitely to my working partner and impeccable editor, Sue Lascelles. Also, a very special thanks to colleague and professional photographer, Anton Zemlyanoy, for his tireless work on ever improving the quality of the photos in this book. Very grateful!

Note to Reader

Dear Reader: Please note that all names have been altered to preserve confidentiality. Permission has been granted by all those whose photographs appear in the text, including the estate of one late colleague. I have permission to reproduce all the images in the book.

Foreword

Dr. Lita Crociani-Windland and Dame Ruth Silver

The foreword to this book has its own natural history: Ruth and Lita first met when Lita was invited to be one of the directors of the Centre for Social Dreaming. When Ruth and Lita were invited to have a conversation with Rose about writing a foreword for the book, an idea found Lita as a willing thinker. The idea was to base the foreword on a dialogue between her and Ruth, rather than having just one author. We all liked that idea. The dialogue form, in having more than one voice, mirrors the importance of connections and the binocular vision[1] embedded in the consultative process of Social Dream Drawing that this book is a guide to. The process, as the reader will see, is based on working with dreams through both words and drawings; the verbal and the visual both have a part to play. Social Dream Drawing involves group work and is profoundly psychosocial in that it has its roots both in psychoanalytically derived practices, such as the use of free association and amplification, and a belief in the social connectedness that links all of us in both conscious and unconscious ways. The book itself encompasses so many different levels that one voice would not be able to do justice to it. Before going any further, however, some further introductions to the writers of this foreword may give readers a sense of why we are here to introduce this book.

Dame Ruth Silver is a clinical psychologist, educationalist and consultant with a long association to Social Dreaming; she worked with Gordon Lawrence, was the founding Chair of the Gordon Lawrence Foundation, with Rose being the patron at the time. Gordon Lawrence was the originator of Social Dreaming as an innovative consultancy process and Ruth is now the patron of the Centre for Social Dreaming, alongside her many other roles, which include having been founding president of the independent think tank *Further Education Trust for Leadership (FETL)*, where Social Dreaming has had its place. Having known of Rose by reputation for a long time, Ruth first really met Rose properly at an ISPSO conference Ruth attended in her role as Chair of the Gordon Lawrence Foundation. She has a strong recollection of Rose engaging in an Oxford debate and was very taken by her capacity to hold her own in a quiet, graceful and yet incisive way. She was the best debater there. Then when Gordon Lawrence died, they had a chance to meet at his funeral. Their professional link is through their attachment to Social Dreaming as a great innovation and helpful way to get to meanings.

Dr. Lita Crociani-Windland is an academic working in Sociology and Psychosocial Studies. She is a board member of the Centre for Social Dreaming and Association for Psychosocial Studies and also co-chair of the Association for Psychoanalysis of Culture and Society. She first met Rose and her husband, Prof. Dr Burkard Sievers, when they ran a workshop at the University of the West of England, where Lita has been based for the last 20 years. The workshop was based on a process that involved the use of drawing to help participants work on a deeper understanding of their work roles. Lita was very impressed by the workshop and in hindsight, the workshop could be seen as a precursor to the current Social Dream Drawing innovation. Somewhat surprisingly for someone already so accomplished, Rose then decided to embark on Doctoral Studies and Lita was asked to be a supervisor for Rose's Doctoral work alongside Anne-Marie Cummins. That marked the beginning of an extremely fruitful and rewarding collaboration, where Lita had the privilege of seeing Social Dream Drawing through initial conception to birth, its development as an academically rigorous research project and now its growth as a fully-fledged practice embraced by others in different parts of the world. What was truly amazing during Rose's doctoral study was her capacity to embrace the student role after having had an extremely accomplished professional consultant position. This is not an easy thing to do: moving from learner to expert is the usual trajectory, but going from expert to learner is uncommon and far harder. Back to binocular vision: Rose was able to be both an expert and a learner, and this speaks to Rose's capacity to hold different perspectives and positions at the same time, something required by the double task of simultaneously developing and researching the development of Social Dream Drawing as a professional and research tool.

In our dialogue, there were lots of 'both and', and this could be seen as a signature for this book. The book presents both a deepening and an extension of the work initiated by Gordon Lawrence's Social Dreaming. Social Dream Drawing has roots in that work while at the same time giving it an additional dimension through the use of drawing. It uses words and images. It has and deploys a social and group dimension and a psychological one in helping individuals work through dilemmas. It is truly a deeply psychosocial innovation, bringing the visual into play in a time when our culture has become increasingly visual and both practices and academic disciplines have had to become more visually and digitally literate. This very accessible book and the practice of Social Dream Drawing fits the world we now live in, where we are continually bombarded by visual information and we need to learn how to work with it. Ruth offered the image of Social Dream Drawing as a dual carriageway offering a way of working inclusively across many barriers, such as a second language or a different educational trajectory to the more traditional one: this way of working can offer a new set of literacies that can be used with some of the people Ruth has championed all her life, marginalised young people and deprived communities, and can allow their creativity expression. The dual carriageway metaphor includes the idea that different speeds are possible, that drawings don't have to be beautiful or accomplished and this she thought could be a useful way of presenting the process to young people.

Social Dream Drawing is a new and exciting tool, joining a set of psychosocial ways of working that can be applied for consultative and research purposes.[2] The book stretches between different theoretical and cultural ways of understanding dreams and the unconscious, founded on rigorous academic study, as well as providing a detailed guide to how to conduct and move through the different phases of Social Dream Drawing. All this multilayered content is given in a very accessible style, giving the reader a sense of why dreams are important, where they fit historically, sociologically, anthropologically, why drawing is useful, how the bodily movement in drawing brings an additional element to working with the dream content. Our hope is that Social Dream Drawing will be used not just in terms of research and consultation work but also in education. Ruth has used Social Dreaming very successfully in educational settings and for educational purposes in the past and this extension of it can also be extremely useful. The book adds to the relatively few in-depth books on Social Dreaming beyond Gordon Lawrence's original work.

What is also remarkable about this book is its generosity in offering such a detailed 'how to' manual aspect that should enable educators, consultants and researchers to add this way of working to their tools to access unconscious dynamics. It marks quite a different attitude to the one that holds things back, instead, it is an invitation to innovate, to try it out and try things out. It does this on the basis of a well-grounded understanding of why and how, of important concepts and their origins and critiques that can help innovation stay within the safe practice. It is encouraging and confidence building in its gesture. One of the real achievements of the book is that it has all the weight of a long and accomplished consultancy career, combined with academic rigour, and yet is able to convey all its content in a clear and accessible style. As Lita noted, this is not the case for most academic books, but the clarity here almost belies the underlying complexity. In this book, it can be said that 'simplicity is complexity resolved' to quote the sculptor Constantin Brancusi. This thought brought us back to the use of drawings and how helpful it is to see that the varying levels of skills in the drawings done by participants has no effect on how meaning is expressed and can be perceived. This is important as many people are very nervous when it comes to drawing, Lita was taken back to a time when she taught painting and led group painting exercises and how terrified some people could be, usually because of bad educational experiences in their past. The drawings and the narratives in this book should be able to reassure the nervous 'non-artists' among us. Nonetheless, we thought Rose was able to make something difficult look easy to do, something great artists can do. And the narratives told of how surprised people could be by what came through their dreams and drawings when helped by others and guided by this carefully constructed way of working. The attention to the setting, the thinking through, the sense of having time, no rush, and the careful stewardship were enviable.

The power of free associative thinking comes through in this work and is something that has been under-utilised until recently but is being rediscovered. Social Dream Drawing and other processes based on free associations are going back to the very start and foundations of psychoanalysis to open it up and renew it. That renewal aims to get beyond the individual unconscious and individual blind spots: the groups are used to get beyond the dyadic therapist/client relationship, bringing in more minds thinking and feeling together, inviting the social dimension into the room. So many literacies are outlined in the book and brought together in Social Dream Drawing. First, they are dealt with more separately and then they are brought back into relation. Maybe the better image here is that of the music conductor who knows each instrument and how to bring each together with others at the right time.

Ruth felt rejuvenated by reading this book, and that made us think of its usefulness to both those new to this social way of working with dreams as well as for those who, like herself, have been working with them since the start of such practice. It is a mature work, dripping with the benefit of experience and a dedication to inquiry, that speaks to Roses's curiosity and joy in a work that drove her to leave no stone unturned. Social Dream Drawing is a process based on collaboration rather than competition, something sorely needed in our times of division and too often polarised and antagonistic views. It was great for Lita and Ruth to be given the opportunity to spend time together talking. In a process similar to what happens in dreaming and drawing, we were able to let our impression and evaluation of this book emerge in a flowing way, different images and aspects emerging as we went along. We hope to have done justice to Roses's work and been able to give voice to its many aspects and complexity, given in such accessible ways. Enjoy the book's clarity, but remember it stands on a base of long professional experience and solid academic foundations of enquiry.

Notes

1 Bion, W.R. (1991) Learning from experience. (Original work published 1962), p. 86. Northvale, NJ: Jason Aronson.
2 Long, S. (2013) *Socioanalytic Methods: Discovering the Hidden in Organisations and Social Systems* (1st ed.). Routledge. https://doi.org/10.4324/9780429480355

Introduction

Are you a professional who is working with people who are:

- Changing careers?
- Moving countries?
- Retiring?
- Getting an advanced degree?
- Seeking challenging new employment?
- Being made redundant?
- Mourning a loss?
- Or going through any other major life transition …

If so, then this is the book for you!

It is fair to say that when we are going through major life transitions, we will very likely face new and unanticipated problems and circumstances. In many cases, there will be no familiar template or past experience for us to draw upon, at least consciously, to help us cope in these situations. Even when our transitions are voluntary, such as deciding to do a doctorate or choosing to move to another country, the unfamiliarity and uncertainty are enormous. And new transitions evoke the unrest and insecurity of previous ones.

Not surprisingly, therefore, people dream quite actively during such transitions. As dream researcher Robert Hoss put it to me in an email: 'Life transitions create quite a lot of vivid, often disturbing dreams and nightmares as we try to re-adjust our inner model of reality and our changing sense of self'.[1] Not only are our dreams more active, but the underlying emotions relating to these major changes become actively alive in the dreamworld.

As contemporary neurological research demonstrates, dreams help us adapt to life and the many challenges it throws at us. Dreams are a way of solving problems and working through emotional issues. And tapping into this problem-solving capacity provides enormous resources.

Social Dream-Drawing (also known as SDD) is a methodology I have developed over a period of years, which extracts the learning from the dream and brings it into consciousness. Drawing itself functions as a sort of

DOI: 10.4324/9780429275647-1

investigative tool, as it gradually – line by line or layer by layer – brings the dream material out into the open.

Not only do drawings access more of the original dream material (and thus make this material more available for use in coping with problems), these drawings can be readily shared with others going through the same difficult life changes. These colourful and expressive drawings bring an otherwise internal experience out into the open and often serve as lifelong mementos of a key time in one's life.

This book is a practical guide to the underlying concepts and the specific use of the SDD method, both as an online and as a face-to-face method of learning. The six basic steps of this method are clearly explained, and advice is given on how to organise and prepare participants for the experience. Guidance on how to facilitate a group emphasises the importance of creating a supportive and safe working environment. There are two chapters devoted to follow-up activities that increase the learnings. A special chapter on conducting SDD online demonstrates how well this method works in the virtual world. The book concludes with examples of other uses of the method, including the author's own deep learning experience.

Discovering the power of Social Dream-Drawing

My own story of dream drawings began in 2003. After a graduate class in which I'd discussed a case involving one of my coaching clients, one of the master's students had a dream about the client whose case I had presented. This student brought the five dream drawings to our next class, shown in Figure 0.1.

In this dream, my client (shown with blue hair) takes me (curly hair) to a muddy lake and tells me that babies have died there. During our class, the student shared the dream with us while pointing to the various drawings that told the story. On the one hand, it was an alarming dream, but on the other hand, the drawings were so detailed and well crafted that they helped guide us as we explored their content.

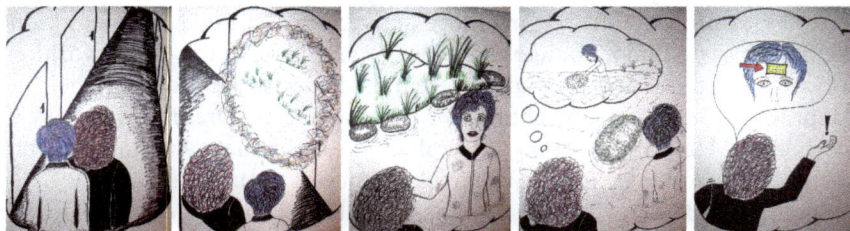

Figure 0.1 Rose and her client

I really didn't know how we could work with these drawings, but using my knowledge of free association, I asked the other students to offer their thoughts and say whatever came to mind. As a result of their comments and my subsequent reflections, I began to recognise aspects of my client that I somehow 'knew' but had never consciously thought about. For example, although she was a paediatrician, she had no children of her own. In addition, she was a client who only wanted to work with me by telephone, and I began to wonder if there hadn't been some very early childhood trauma at the base of that need. And if so, it would not be appropriate to confront her with that.

The associations to these dream pictures provided a kind of 'third eye' on the consultation and opened a great deal of new inner space for me to work with my client, not in the sense of sharing this experience with her, but in the sense of being able to develop and hold more hypotheses about her and her inner world. This experience reaffirmed me in my professional role and re-invigorated my consultation work with my client. And understandably, I became quite excited about the possibilities of exploring drawings of dreams for future work.

I thought of this dream as being a 'social' dream, in the sense that the student dreamt this dream on behalf of my consultation with my client, as opposed to its being a personal dream about her own internal world. This was confirmed by her decision to bring these drawings to the group the following week.

Building on the experience of Social Dreaming

During the years before this experience, I had hosted a number of Social Dreaming workshops. Social Dreaming is a method based on the idea that dreams can have a social aspect as well as a personal aspect. And when people come together to share their dreams, more of the social 'unconscious' of that group can be illuminated. This work can often help a group understand its underlying conflicts and dynamics and lead to solutions for them.

Using Social Dreaming as a model, I began working with small groups of colleagues and students in the Netherlands and in Germany to test whether dream drawings could be a valuable resource. In 2009, I began my doctoral studies in the United Kingdom, and my goal was to test the usefulness of this way of working with a broader selection of participants. My doctoral advisors suggested I run an SDD group composed of native English speakers, so I worked with one group in London and another in Bristol. My findings demonstrated that the principal usefulness of this method, which I had now refined, was to help people going through major life changes. In SDD, I had developed a tool that professionals in many different fields could use to help such people.

The purpose of this book

This book is designed to be a useful manual for anyone who is potentially interested in using SDD with their clients, students or colleagues.

Chapters 1–3 cover the underlying theory for this method. Chapter 1, 'How dreams help us', summarises current neurological research on the importance of dreams and offers an integrated theory of dreaming drawn from a number of different theorists. This chapter emphasises the creative and problem-solving aspects of working with dreams during uncertain times.

Chapter 2, 'The advantages and challenges of drawing one's dreams', considers the importance of the physical act of drawing a dream and its link to the physical experience of dreaming. It cites research that demonstrates drawing a dream produces more original dream material than just a verbal telling. The value of a physical reminder (i.e. the dream drawing itself), representing a deeply meaningful time in one's life, is also emphasised.

Chapter 3, 'The support and learning from group work', explores how, in many difficult life situations, working with and participating in groups of like-minded people can have a healing and motivating effect. It describes how group participants bring insights of their own to the dreams of others that add a major source of new learning. Common issues are identified and mutual support increases.

The next section, Chapters 4–7, contains practical information on all aspects of undertaking the SDD method. Chapter 4, 'Organising and undertaking a Social Dream-Drawing workshop', describes in detail the preparatory steps for organising such a workshop, including identifying a theme, assembling a group, rules for confidentiality and finding an appropriate venue. I will be offering advice on the number of workshops to offer and which dream drawings one accepts, and which not.

Chapter 5, 'Conducting a Social Dream-Drawing workshop', describes in detail the six specific steps in an SDD workshop. The chapter opens with an extensive discussion of how the room itself should be prepared for each session.

Chapters 6 and 7 offer suggested activities to extend the learning beyond the workshop itself. Chapter 6, 'The final review session', focuses on facilitating the individual learning from the workshop. Chapter 7, 'Extended integration of Social Dream-Drawing learning', looks at the group learning from an SDD workshop and is especially appropriate for groups of co-workers whose own group dynamics are central to their effective work.

Chapter 8, 'The role of facilitator', is of central importance to anyone conducting an SDD workshop themselves. People often approach this work with a degree of anxiety. Because of the intimate material of the dreams and the sense of safety a group needs to work with this material, I offer key suggestions for facilitating the group in a safe and containing way. Normal anxieties about sharing dream material and drawings are central to how facilitators run these groups, and specific strategies for dealing with concerns and challenges will be described in order to create a safe and creative working environment.

The content of Chapter 9 has been forced upon us by world events. In response to the need to work online, this chapter, 'Coronavirus and working online', describes a workshop done in 2021 on Zoom. The method worked extremely well, as is detailed in the chapter.

Chapter 10, 'Other ways of using Social Dream-Drawing', describes four different new ways SDD has been used by colleagues of mine and by myself. The book concludes with an example of my own personal experience of SDD.

Throughout this book, you will find dream drawings and testimonies from people who have participated in SDD groups. All names have been changed to protect confidentiality. They identify how this experience helped them through their own personal transitions, which include moving from one country to another, starting a new job, bereavement, doing a doctorate and retirement.

My great hope in writing this book for you, dear reader, is that you will, like so many others besides me, catch the bug of excitement at the profound and amazing experience that SDD can be.

Note

1   Hoss, R. (2019) Private email correspondence.

Chapter 1

How dreams help us

There's no doubt that dreams can be a powerful source of help and inspiration in our lives. In various fields and throughout the world, contemporary and historical examples abound. Here are a few famous ones:

- Paul McCartney woke up from a dream where the melody and the key to his masterpiece 'Yesterday' had come to him. He went directly to his piano and figured out the chords. He wanted to capture it before it disappeared.[1]
- In 1816, Mary Godwin (soon to be Mary Shelley) had a frightening dream about a monster created by a scientist. This monster, whom we now know as Frankenstein, would eventually believe that it was a god with power over all others.
- Albert Einstein cited two dreams that served as the inspiration for one of the most famous theories of all time, his theory of relativity. One dream was about a dispute with a farmer concerning electrified cows, and in the other, he was falling uncontrolled down a mountainside. The faster he went, the more the stars above were changing.

These dreams and many more have served as inspirations to many famous people. All of us can probably cite similar examples in our own lives.

And lest we imagine that this is just a contemporary phenomenon, it is important to bear in mind that these exotic, powerful and puzzling night-time events have engaged and fascinated people since the beginning of time. Since dreaming first began, primitive societies, theorists and scientists have sought to understand them and create meaning from them. A major part of this quest has been to use dreams as a resource for understanding peoples' lives and daily realities. This quest continues to this day. I would agree with Tavistock consultant David Armstrong's observation:

> I do not see dreams as containers of meaning – a puzzle to be solved once and for all; but rather as containers for meaning; available narratives through which we negotiate and seek formulation for the emotional experiences we register.[2]

DOI: 10.4324/9780429275647-2

At the beginning ...

Long before psychoanalysis located dreaming in the individual and way before contemporary neurological research identified the area of the brain from where dreams emanate, dreams were seen as visitations from powerful and unknown external sources. Throughout the ancient world, dreams were thought to facilitate a direct connection to figures in the spiritual world, and they were incorporated into significant religious and cultural rituals. This dream material would offer what Matthew Walker, University of California Professor of Neuroscience and author of the best-selling book *Why We Sleep*, refers to as 'information divine' to guide them in their decision-making and daily routines.[3]

Belief that dreams provide important guidance is found in all major world religions. In the biblical tradition, for example, God communicated to his prophets through dreams. The most famous is Jacob's dream of a ladder, which symbolised the connection between heaven and earth, man and God. At the time God visited Jacob, he was experiencing a crisis of strength and courage. In the dream, God repeats his promise to safeguard a homeland for the descendants of Abraham and Isaac (Genesis: 12–15). The dream gave Jacob strength and made him more courageous.[4]

In Islam, there is the 'great tradition of the spiritual dream',[5] most notably Mohammed's famous dream (or revelation), the Night Journey. In this dream, Angel Gabriel takes Mohammed from his small life in Mecca to the centre of the world (what is now the Temple Mount in Jerusalem). This dream was, for Mohammed, a confirmation that he was destined to be a messenger from God, who occupied the seat of absolute power and knowledge.

In both these examples, dreams and the messages they brought from an external power gave these men in crisis the strength to continue and the conviction of their beliefs. No wonder they are now enshrined in these religious traditions.

Where today, we might view the contents of these dreams metaphorically, in times gone by, they were believed to be true omens. Dreams were believed to bring wisdom from those more powerful than us and guide us. They brought reassurance and security to cope with the dangers and threats of the external world.

Dreams begin with us

All of these beliefs about dreams and many more were known to Sigmund Freud, who was an avid student of ancient civilisations and actively collected historical artefacts. By the time of his death in 1939, he had a huge collection of reproductions and originals from such ancient kingdoms as Egypt, Greece, Rome, India, China and Eritrea. He was particularly fascinated with Egyptian hieroglyphs, which he compared to the content of dreams.

Freud was well aware of ancient practices relating to dreaming. Former research fellow at the Sigmund Freud Institute in Frankfurt, Christine Walde, quotes him as saying: 'I think that in general it is a good plan occasionally to bear in mind the fact that people were in the habit of dreaming before there was such a thing as psychoanalysis'.[6]

Freud more or less changed history by being the first to locate dreams in the psychic life of the dreamer. No more external forces entering the passive human system. The dreams emanate from us. And they are very significant events.

In addition to locating dreams within us, he also formulated the theory that they emanated from our unconscious, a part of ourselves that exists well below the surface of conscious awareness. Freud viewed the material in our unconscious as having an enormous impact on our behaviour and feelings. But, according to him, this important material is almost impossible to access. At times, it is revealed in slips of the tongue or in strange physical symptoms. And also, it is revealed in our dreams.

From Freud's perspective, dreams were a gold mine of material through which he could examine the unconscious repressions of his patients and their accompanying neuroses. Freud's famous statement that *Dreams are the royal road to the unconscious*, has since entered the mainstream. Freud, in developing the practice and theory of psychoanalysis, maintained that accessing these processes beyond awareness in order to learn what is influencing our feelings and behaviours would eventually allow us to modify our lives for the better.

Despite this revolutionary contribution to the notion of dream studies, Freud's perspective on how dreams help us has now largely been superseded by further theorists. In brief, Freud's notion is that dreams help us because they protect us from the negative and taboo wishes and desires that we truly hold but that are absolutely unacceptable to acknowledge. Because they are not socially and personally acceptable, we repress them. We store and hide all our unwanted desires and wishes in our unconscious, a dark and scary place.

Freud thought dreams functioned as a release valve for these taboo instincts and desires as well as a means of disguising them. Their confusing and illogical material (what he termed 'manifest content') disguises their true content ('latent content') so that dreamers do not have to be confronted with them. Therefore, the purpose of dreaming is to protect the dreamer from waking up with a jolt and being confronted with these repressed desires.

While Freud's notion that dreams were disguising unmet needs and desires repressed in the unconscious has since been revised, one lasting contribution to working with dreams has been his development of free association (a method used in Social Dream-Drawing and discussed in detail in Chapter 3). Free association, which encourages the patient to say whatever comes to mind, without censorship, still serves as a cornerstone to dream work. As summarised by contemporary psychoanalyst Christopher Bollas: 'The method of free association gains access to this infinite of meaning, to a world of thinking and of communicating that is entirely out of consciousness'.[7] In this way, Freud developed the practice of psychoanalysis, the goal of which is to help patients gain an understanding of what lies under the surface of their ordinary awareness, which often wreaks so much havoc in their waking lives.

The development of other perspectives on the nature of the unconscious and the function of dreaming began most notably with Freud's younger contemporary, C. J. Jung. As opposed to functioning as a disguise, dreams are, from Jung's perspective 'a part of nature'.[8] He saw the dream as a normal, spontaneous and creative expression of the unconscious.

Jung also believed that dreams were visual, and he himself drew many of his own dreams, most notably in the recently uncovered *Red Book*.[9] Other theorists have expanded and supported Jung's perspective, and it is this view of dreaming and the nature of the unconscious that underlies the practice of Social Dream-Drawing (also known as SDD).

This notion of a creative unconscious is reflected in the dream drawing below by Christine, a German participant in an SDD workshop. When she made the drawing, she was a professor approaching retirement from the university where she had worked for 27 years. Her drawing (see Figure 1.1) shows herself admiring two people fleeing a red brick building – '*schöner alter Backstein*' – on old-fashioned bicycles. This building reminded her of the old bakehouses in the part of Germany where she grew up.

For Christine, this dream drawing expressed the split she experienced between her true creative professional self (on the bicycles) and her university (the redbrick bakehouse). In a sense, this dream drawing is a form of self-portrait since it portrays two conflicting sides of herself. One side is the creative and playful Christine. The other side is the hardworking and serious Christine.

She saw the university as interfering with her creativity and her students as being a constant source of disappointment. During the course of the group's associations to her drawing, however, she began to realise, that, in fact, over the course of her career, her university had actually given her great freedom to work creatively.

In my follow-up interview with her a few years later, she said that she began to realise that her institution had given her a great deal of leeway in creating new programmes and that some of her students had really benefitted from this. Over the course of the workshops, she gained a more balanced perspective on the esteem in which she was held by her institution and the benefits and opportunities it had offered her. So the initial problem of feeling stymied by the system morphed into a more realistic assessment of the situation.

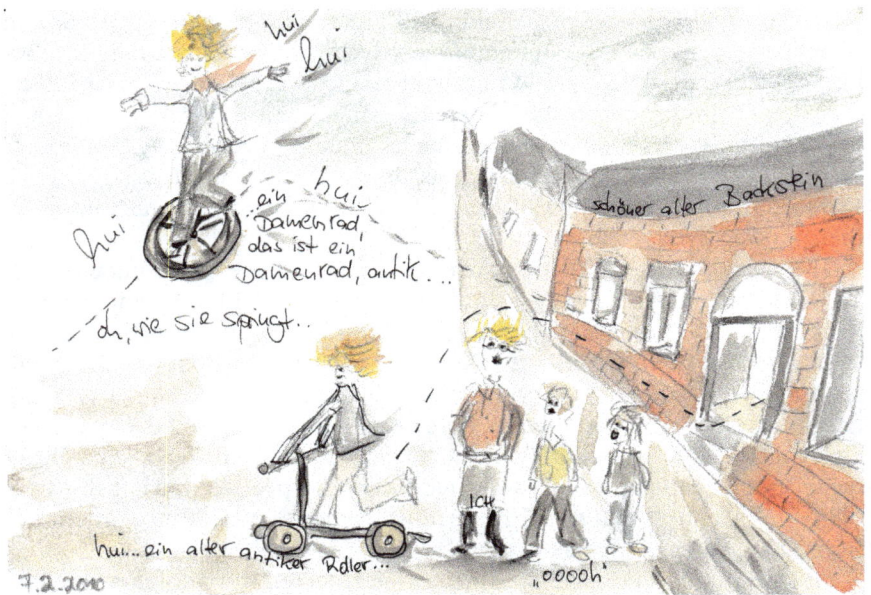

Figure 1.1 Red brick bakehouse

As a result, she was able to appreciate how much she really was valued by her institution and the benefit and opportunities it had offered her. She was now able to find a renewed enthusiasm for her university work, which would represent her last creative efforts as a professor. She decided to delay her retirement plans. Eventually, she would be able to leave her professional home in a positive way.

How can dreams help us, especially during transitions?

Our ancient ancestors, in their attempts to cope with the challenges relating to their survival and success as societies, developed various ways of making use of their dream experiences to guide their decision-making. Long before the contemporary neurological confirmation of the problem-solving value of dreaming, ancient societies used these external visitations to resolve important dilemmas.

One good example involved the Native American Crow Indian tribe, living in the Yellowstone River Valley in the nineteenth century. As a practice, whenever they faced a difficult situation, they sent out selected tribe members, usually young men or boys, who were called dream-seekers, to the wilderness. Their task was to 'plead for the Great Spirit to grant a dream'.[10] After a dream came, the elders would interpret it in relation to their current problem.

In the 1850s, the Crow were faced with imminent destruction by white settlers and soldiers, who were crowding them out of their native lands and killing off their beloved buffaloes. The tribe sent out a nine-year-old boy named Petty Coups to facilitate the tribe's 'response to their longer term fate at the hands of the whites'.[11] Petty's subsequent dream included images of the buffalo being replaced by 'spotted buffalo'.[12] The spotted buffalo image in the dream was interpreted as being the white man's cow. This, in turn, was interpreted as relating to the reality of the future, as former hunting lands were increasingly being taken over as grazing pastures for the bulls and cows of the white man. The elders concluded that they must come to terms with this future rather than resist it in the way that many other Indian tribes had, particularly the Sioux and the Blackfoot. This led them to negotiate terms that, while not insuring that they kept their traditional hunting life, allowed them to survive as a tribe.

The idea that dreams are valuable in solving problems in our daily life – even problems that are not yet in our consciousness – has been confirmed over and over again by contemporary theorists and neurological researchers. As Matthew Walker points out: 'Little wonder, then, that you have never been told to "stay awake on a problem". Instead, you are instructed to "sleep on it"'.[13]

There are many factors to account for this.

To begin with, there is the notion that there is an ongoing connection between the waking self and the sleeping self, in the sense that our conscious thoughts have a continuous connection with those of our dreams. As such, as the contemporary psychoanalyst Christopher Bollas puts it, 'the night self begins *knowingly* to dream *for* the day self'.[14] Just as it is said that the analytic patient brings dreams specifically for his analyst, one can say that the dreaming self offers its creations to the conscious self in order to contribute to the dreamer's well-being. And from Bollas's perspective, this allows the two parts to work in 'partnership'.[15]

How do dreams work?

Robert Hoss, dream researcher and author, puts it very simply. He argues that the process that dreams help us with is to adapt to life, whatever challenges and problems it throws at us. As he writes, these dreams have 'the aim of problem solving and, in the process, learning how to better deal with adverse life situations, physical and emotional threats as well as conflicted or impactful social situations'.[16] Naturally then, the more extreme and difficult the problems are, the more dreams can be a resource for creative adapting and problem-solving.

So how does this work?

Contemporary science has shown us that dreams emerge from the associative cortex of the brain that is involved with emotional memory processing and consolidation. Dreams transform problems from the conscious into another form, the form of a dream. This reactivation process is seen by some researchers as a rehearsal scenario of the current problem. In our dreams, we practise different solutions to these troubling issues in a safe space and then eventually integrate or reject their content depending on the outcome of the dream.

In fact, building on Freud's famous phrase, psychiatrist and Gestalt founder Fritz Perls calls dreams 'the royal road to integration',[17] as they enable us to become whole by reclaiming the alienated parts of our personality. This process of integrating what has previously been denied or separate takes place in a very particular way in our dream world. As Hoss writes:

> This type of dream metaphorically pictures an adverse event in waking life and introduces and tests various problem solving or resolution scenarios in order to learn how better to deal with that life situation and future situations like it. This seems to be the most common problem resolution dream. Observing the resolution scenarios can provide valuable insight or clues as to how the dreamer might proceed in waking life. This is particularly true when the scenario or outcome in the dream is emotionally reinforced (rewarded with a positive ending).[18]

New pieces of information are synthesised with pre-existing knowledge. As a result, we become inspired to seek alternative ways to handle new situations, using the 'new forms of creative insight'[19] provided by the dreams.

Now, as we all know, the forms of our dreams are often completely mysterious and confusing, which doesn't make it easy for us to make use of them. That is exactly why I have developed SDD: to help people going through big life changes make use of their dreams.

Why is dream material so confusing?

One can refer again to Freud's position that dream material is intentionally confusing in order to protect the dreamer from deeper feelings. Psychoanalyst Montague Ullman notes this 'makes possible the containment of terror and impulse by the decorum of art and symbolism'.[20] Thus, he continues, 'the dream recapitulates and states more than the individual can absorb into his immediate waking experience'.[21]

Dreams, unlike our waking thoughts, are not restrained by the logic and realism that we face in our everyday lives. As Walker explains, during REM sleep, 'the brain becomes actively biased toward seeking out the most distant, nonobvious links between sets of information'[22] in service of the process of coping with daytime problems. It becomes a kind of creative search engine, seeking connections and themes linking aspects of our biography that relate to our current preoccupations and concerns.

Walker describes it this way:

> Like an insightful interview, dreaming takes the approach of interro-
> gating our recent autobiographical experience and skillfully position-
> ing it within the context of past experiences and accomplishments,
> building a rich tapestry of meaning 'How can I understand and connect
> that which I have recently learnt with that I already know, and in doing
> so, discover insightful new links and revelations?' Moreover, 'What
> have I done in the past that might be useful in potentially solving this
> newly experienced problem in the future?'.... REM sleep, and the act of
> dreaming, takes that which we have learnt in one experience setting and
> seeks to apply it to others stored in memory.[23]

So dreaming builds on our strengths and what we know from experience.

All major life transitions involve uncertainty and anxiety, even those we
have chosen to make. In these uncertain periods, people dream quite actively,
and there are important reasons for that. Walker notes that 'between 35 and
55 percent of emotional themes and concerns that participants were having while they were awake during the day powerfully and unambiguously
resurfaced in the dreams they were having at night'.[24] This means that, as
confusing as it is, dream material often relates directly to current emotional
daytime concerns and themes.

However, in the dream state, this material is worked with in a very different
way than in our conscious state. According to Walker, there is a strong decrease
in a key stress-inducing chemical, noradrenaline, during REM sleep.[25] Because
of that, the daytime worrying material is somehow disarmed and reframed in
the context of a more relaxed mental state. Thus, as Walker puts it: 'REM-sleep
dreaming offers a form of overnight therapy .... [it] takes the painful sting out of
difficult, even traumatic, emotional episodes you have experienced during the
day, offering emotional resolution when you awake the next morning'.[26]

So the stressful memories from our daily life are reconfigured in such a
way as to reduce their stressful impact. But this is just the dreaming part.
There is more.

The research of Rosalie Cartwright, Professor Emeritus of Rush
University Medical Center's Graduate Neuroscience Division (Chicago),
shows that dreaming's ability to help us cope with difficult situations is
directly dependent on the content of the dreams themselves. Simply put,
the more the material in the dream is directly connected to the 'emotional
themes and sentiments of the waking trauma',[27] the more therapeutic impact
it has. As Walker notes, 'REM sleep is necessary but not sufficient. It is both
the act of dreaming and the associated content of those dreams that deter-
mine creative success'.[28]

At various times in our lives, many of us will go through a natural set
of life transitions, i.e. childhood, adolescence, marriage, parenting, midlife

and approaching death. Dream researcher Alan Siegel has noted that during each of these transition times, dream material is present relating to the emotions underlying that change in life.[29]

When going through more extreme transitions, however, such as starting a new job or moving from one country to another, our dreams are not only more active, but also the underlying emotions relating to these big changes come actively alive in the dreamworld.

Figure 1.2 shows a dream drawing representing both types of transitions: those that are a normal part of life and those that are especially fraught with uncertainty and change.

Martin was taking up a new position as a university lecturer after being a full-time psychotherapist. He brought the above drawing – with images from two different dreams that he had had three days apart – to an SDD workshop held in Santiago, Chile, in 2009. The theme of this workshop was 'What do I risk in my work?' (The following accounts of his dreams are based on the original transcripts of the workshop.)

On the left, Martin depicts a fragment from a dream he had the day after learning about the theme of the workshop. In the dream, he sees himself facing forward and then views himself from above. He has plenty of hair on both sides of his head and at the front, but he has almost none, or just fuzz, on the top of his head. When looking at himself face-on, he didn't realise at first that he had lost his hair. This happened only when he looked at himself from above or from behind. He then developed a feeling of anxiety and

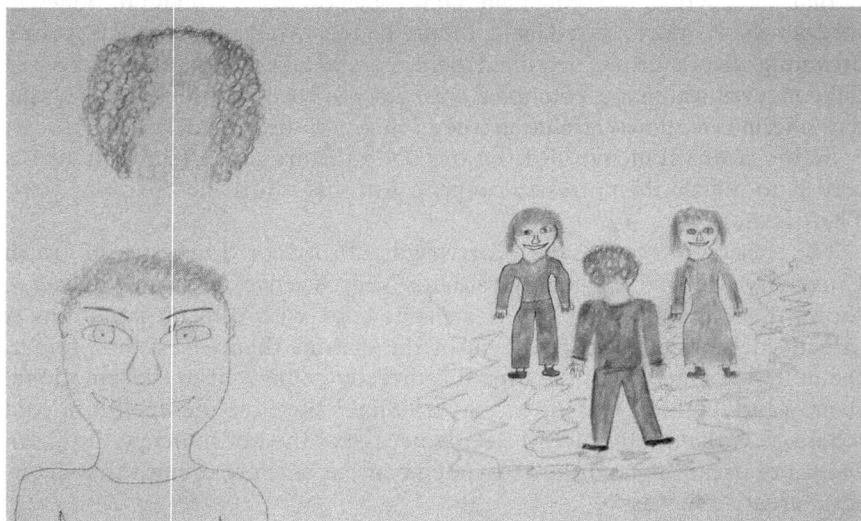

Figure 1.2 New professor with alopecia

distress since he had not been able to tell what was happening to him when looking at himself face-on.

The second fragment (on the right) relates to a dream Martin had three days after the first one. In this dream, he sees three female students who, at the end of class, approach him and remark on how interesting the lesson was. While this takes place, he realises he has forgotten to put on his belt and his trousers are falling down. This generates distress but also produces an erotic feeling.

The first dream can be seen as an anxiety dream relating to becoming truly middle aged, also represented by taking on the prominent role of a professor. Martin related the baldness at the top of his head to the condition of alopecia, an illness his father had.

The second dream (and drawing) can be seen as relating to the major life change of starting a new career and taking on a senior position at a major university. Going from self-employment to full-time work in an organisation is not an easy life transition. This change evoked in Martin strong anxieties relating specifically to the role of professor. As noted in the transcript of the session, his associations to the second dream 'refer to a sense of eroticism and the seduction of others, especially women, in his role of professor'.

In the reflection session, which is part of every SDD workshop, Martin identified two major risks related to these drawings. One is the risk that his work will make him unhealthy (losing hair). He saw that he had to endeavour to strike a healthy balance between his work and personal life. The other is the risk of being perceived as irrelevant or unable to succeed in a new role. One can feel totally naked in such circumstances.

In a follow-up interview a year and a half later, Martin recognised even more clearly how significant a time this had been for him. What connected the two drawings was his difficult experience of transitioning from full-time clinical practice to being a business school professor. Not only was it 'very difficult in terms of the students and how to connect with them' and the 'process of finding a role as a teacher', but there were also strongly erotic aspects to this work. He felt 'trapped … in this seductive role'.

The drawing of these two dreams and working on them with the group helped him recognise the impact of these two simultaneously difficult experiences. From his new perspective after the passage of time, he had now made this transition. The work on his dream drawings was very helpful for him in recognising the frightening implications of the stress he was under at the time.

Dreams and our well-being

One can certainly say that nothing much has changed about dreaming since we first began to do it. What has evolved, however, is a greater understanding of why we dream and how the act of dreaming and then further work with dream material can help us adapt to life's problems and challenges.

As a species, we have always endeavoured to relate and make use of these puzzling dream experiences. First considered visitations from external powers, dreams are now known to emanate from our unconscious. Once considered (by Freud) to function as protections against our taboo desires, they are now recognised for their extraordinary creative and problem-solving capacities.

As such, we can confidently say that dreams can act as a major resource for our well-being.

Notes

1　Walker, M. (2017) *Why We Sleep: The New Science of Sleep and Dreams*. UK: Penguin, p. 221.
2　Armstrong, D. (1996) The recovery of meaning. Paper presented to the annual symposium of the International Society for the Psychoanalytic Study of Organizations, 'Organisation 2000: Psychoanalytic Perspectives', June 1996, New York.
3　Walker, M. (2017) *Why We Sleep: The New Science of Sleep and Dreams*. UK: Penguin, p. 199.
4　The Companion Bible (1974) Grand Rapids: Zondervan Bible Publishers, p. 41.
5　Coxhead, D. and Hiller, S. (1976) *Dreams: Visions of the Night*. New York: Thames and Hudson, p. 9.
6　Walde, C. (1999) Dream interpretation in a prosperous age? In: Shulman, D. and Stroumsa, G.G., eds., *Dream Cultures: Explorations in the Comparative History of Dreaming*. New York: Oxford University Press, p. 121.
7　Bollas, C. (2011) *The Christopher Bollas Reader*. London: Routledge, p. 251.
8　Jung, C.G. (1961) *Memories, Dreams, Reflections*. Reprint. London: Fontana, 1995, p. 185.
9　Jung, C.G. (1930) *The Red Book: Liber Novus*. Reprint. New York: The Philemon Foundation & W.W. Norton & Co., 2009.
10　Gosling, J. and Case, P. (2013) Social dreaming and ecocentric ethics: sources of non-rational insight in the face of climate change catastrophe. *Organization*. 20 (5), p. 711.
11　Ibid.
12　Ibid., p. 712.
13　Walker, M. (2017) *Why We Sleep: The New Science of Sleep and Dreams*. UK: Penguin, p. 229.
14　Bollas, C. (2011) *The Christopher Bollas Reader*. London: Routledge, p. 254.
15　Ibid.
16　Hoss, R. (2019b) *Dream Language: A Handbook for Dreamwork* (2nd edition). (PDF version), p.102. Ashland, Oregon, USA: Innersource.
17　Perls, F. (1970) Dream seminars. In: Fagan, J. and Shepherd, I.L., eds., *Gestalt Therapy Now*. New York: Harper & Row.
18　Hoss, R. (2019b) *Dream Language: A Handbook for Dreamwork* (2nd edition). (PDF version), p. 222. Ashland, Oregon, USA: Innersource.
19　Bollas, C. (2011) *The Christopher Bollas Reader*. London: Routledge, p. 257.
20　Ullman, M. (1960) The social roots of the dream. *The American Journal of Psychoanalysis*. 20, p. 182.
21　Ibid., p. 183.
22　Walker, M. (2017) *Why We Sleep: The New Science of Sleep and Dreams*. UK: Penguin, p. 226.

23 Ibid., p. 231.
24 Ibid., p. 204.
25 Ibid., p. 208.
26 Ibid., p. 207.
27 Ibid., p. 211.
28 Ibid., pp. 226–7.
29 Schredl, M. (2019) Typical dream themes. In: Hoss, R, Valli, K. and Gongloff, R., eds., *Dreams: Understanding Biology, Psychology, and Culture.* Volume 1. Santa Barbara: ABC-CLIO, p. 187.

Chapter 2

The advantages and challenges of drawing one's dreams

When we mention to others that we have dreamt something important, often their first response is the question: 'Did you write it down?' In our Western culture, there is the general idea that the best and only way to make sense of our dreams (as if one can actually make sense of them) is to write them down as soon as possible.

This notion of putting dreams into words began with Freud and his monumental 1900 publication *The Interpretation of Dreams*.[1] For him telling dreams was the best (and only) way to work with them. This is rather ironic because Freud himself was a prolific and passionate drawer, being fascinated with Egyptian hieroglyphics and other visual media. His office was strewn with photographs and replicas of ancient sculptures. In his time, German researchers considered drawing instrumental to scientific discovery, and, in Freud's earlier roles of biologist and scientist, his scientific drawings, so to say, 'put him on the map' as an esteemed scientist.

Despite this passion, and although he noted that images were closer to the unconscious than writing, Freud nevertheless favoured the 'talking' rather than the 'drawing' cure. Freud believed that it was only through words (i.e. word-presentations) that data would come to consciousness, rather than the more sensual images, which would comprise the drawings of dreams. Despite the fact that he did not work with dream drawings, Freud often acknowledged that dreams were primarily visual in content.

Freud's preference for the talking cure is particularly ironic because one of his most famous cases involved a patient named Pankejeff, whom he called the Wolf Man. Early in his analysis with Freud, Pankejeff verbally shared a dream of five wolves standing in a tree outside his bedroom window and then showed Freud his drawing of this dream. While it is not known whether Freud had asked for a drawing or whether the patient had offered it of his own volition, it is clear that this drawing catalysed the treatment process and Freud's own theoretical developments in a major way. In this respect, I consider Freud's famous case of the Wolf Man to be the very first Social Dream-Drawing workshop.

DOI: 10.4324/9780429275647-3

Various psychoanalysts and researchers have explored and written about the use of dream drawings.[2] The most well-known of these is Carl Jung, who believed firmly that dreams were visual. Jung drew many of his own dreams, mostly notably in the recently uncovered *Red Book*.[3] I think it is fair to say, perhaps because of Freud's own prejudice, that this work sits largely outside the mainstream of ongoing psychoanalytic practice.

Contemporary practitioners utilise various ways of accessing dream material, including not just drawing but also dramatising and sculpting their content. These techniques function as 'an outside agent in helping the dreamer to discover the inward journey of self interpreting the dream',[4] as does Social Dream-Drawing.

As mentioned in Chapter 1, a dream is a message from the unconscious and, thus, by definition, it has a meaning. What this message is and what the deeper meaning may be are pretty much impossible to discern at the time, and these aspects are generally considered to require some sort of verbal therapeutic or group experience for further illumination.

What has been discovered in research on dreaming, both by myself and others, however, is that making a visual representation of the dream experience is of great benefit for a number of reasons.

The physical reanimation of the dream

However one thinks about what a dream is and what it means, we know that it emanates from the body. It comes from within our bodies. As a matter of fact, very often, dreamers wake up with the residual physical sensation in their bodies relating to what they have dreamt. Therefore, in the physical act of drawing this night-time event, the bodily aspects of the dreaming experience are revived. They are revived in the movement of the hand and in the observation of the seeing eye. The body is attempting to somehow represent what the inner eye 'saw'.

The hand is one of our most important body parts in terms of representing and acting. It takes. It signals. It holds. It expresses who we are in countless ways. It even types this book. It is active in relating us to the wider world. And at the beginning of our lives, it often functions as a source of comfort and security when we suck our thumbs or fingers.

Richard Serra, the great sculptural artist, has pointed out that the word 'drawing' is itself both an object and a verb.[5] So what we are talking about here is drawing a drawing. There is a physical act linked to a physical experience, and there is an object created by this physical act. As Van Alphen notes: 'The act of drawing is no longer present in the form of the product alone – a likeness – but it is also present as activity'.[6] The physical act of drawing a dream, therefore, itself revitalises the original sensory material experienced during the dream. As such, the drawn object helps the drawer remain connected to the original physical and sensual dream experience.

In this revitalising action, one is not only representing an inner visual, but, in fact, discovering something by making it visible to the physical world. Drawing itself functions as a sort of investigative tool, as it gradually – line by line or layer by layer – brings the dream material out into the open.

Accessing dream material from a regressed state

Freud noted that being in a state of regression fosters the capacity for dreaming, and the act of drawing a dream returns the dreamer to this previous regressive state. Therefore, a second advantage to drawing a dream is the way in which this act brings one back to the dreaming state.

That this state of regression occurs when drawing a dream was confirmed by Stefan Hau, a researcher at the Freud Institute in Frankfurt, Germany. In his fascinating 2004 book, *Träume zeichnen: Über die visuelle Darstellung von Traumbildern* [*Dream Drawings: the visual depiction/picture of dream drawings*],[7] he describes his extensive research on the drawings of dreams by sleepers woken up during REM sleep. Hau made the important discovery that these drawings contain visual patterns associated with children's drawings. They often show either barely sketched or isolated stick figures, with no contextual or background illustration.[8] There are rare references to ground or skylines and a lack of facial features. When analysed, they show an average drawing skill typical of an eight-and-a-half-year-old child.[9]

Therefore, one can say that the act of drawing a dream brings one back to a primitive, childlike state. In fact, as Sapochnik notes, '[d]rawing, because of its connection with motor muscular impulses, is connected with primitive functioning',[10] as is dreaming, with its primitive content.

My experience with dream drawings is consistent with Hau's research. As you look through this book and note the various dream drawings, you will see that they all have this childlike aspect to them, even though, unlike Hau's participants, the people who drew them were not woken out of REM sleep. Perhaps some pictures are better drawn than others due to the innate talent of the artists, but the basic childlike quality is consistent. They evoke the creations that children themselves make, often with the same kinds of crayons and markers, thus conjuring up images of a childish enterprise. The one-off dream leads to a distinct one-off drawing.

Drawing produces more original dream material

Hau discovered that when his subjects drew their dreams, they regressed to an earlier childhood state, which was reflected in the images they drew. In and of itself, this would not be so significant were it not for his further finding. He discovered when comparing the dream drawing to the verbal retelling of the same dream, that, in fact, the drawings contained more original dream material. He concluded, therefore, that the regressive experience of drawing put the dreamer in greater contact with the original sensory experience of the dream and that drawings of dreams capture primitive regressive elements in a more convincing way than just by verbalisation. That said, however, his ultimate conclusion was that the very best way to share dreams was a combination of drawing and telling. It is not an either-or.

Hau's findings are confirmed by Charles Fischer, a psychiatrist at Mount Sinai Hospital in New York. In his treatment of patients, he found that the pictures his patients draw of their dreams evoke images that would otherwise not come to awareness. He writes:

> It is an interesting feature of these experiments that some of the latent content of the dream emerges and becomes evident through the process of drawing the dream. It is very likely that this content would not become evident if the dreams were reported only verbally and not drawn .... There is no doubt that because dreams are largely visual in structure the usual purely verbal analysis results in the overlooking of significant latent content.[11]

Toni, a participant in my research group in Bristol, makes this process very clear. To her, drawing a dream is 'engaging' and often brings back dream material that one had forgotten. She found that the act of drawing a dream ('something from my mind to paper') somehow made the dream 'more solid' and jogged her to remember more details. It was a process of new discovery. After drawing, she found herself regarding the picture and noting: 'That looks right on paper'.

So why is it that more original dream material becomes available when drawing a dream? It is interesting to reflect on why this is the case.

It seems that one important reason has to do with the strict demands of verbalisation. In his classic book *Visual Thinking,* Rudolf Arnheim extensively articulates the difference between language and drawing. He points out that words suggest permanency and stand for a 'fixed concept'.[12] He further notes that '[t]he function of language is essentially conservative and stabilizing, and therefore it also tends, negatively, to make cognition static and immobile'.[13] Words can 'help to freeze notions'.[14] Words function as a kind of 'shell' which are used 'to package ... thoughts for preservation and communication'.[15] Thus one could say that words may often fail to capture the inarticulate, inchoate and confusing dream material.

In addition to the symbolic and constraining function of the verbal, Arnheim notes the linearity of verbal telling. One word, one phrase, one statement comes after another in a sequence that, to the verbaliser, must make sense to the others to whom he or she is talking. They go in one direction. As such, '[v]erbal language is a one-dimensional string of words because it is used by intellectual thinking to label sequences of concepts'.[16] Each word, each statement, is amended by the next into something closer to the intended total meaning. As Langer puts it: 'words have a linear, discrete, successive order; they are strung one after another like beads on a rosary'.[17]

Although a drawing is created in a successive way. i.e. one draws one image after another, very often in an associative way, the drawer is not under the constraint of composing a sentence, which must follow specific rules regarding the sequence of letters and grammar. The sequence of the drawn dream images is not as strictly determined as the sequence of letters and words when writing a sentence. In fact, elements can be erased, moved around or altogether transformed as the dreamer attempts to capture the dream material in more and more detail.

Some argue that verbalising a dream does it a disservice. Philosophy professor Christine Walde notes: 'When dream images, usually consisting of pictures, are transformed into language, the interpreter is already working with a mediated and rationalized construct'. And 'translating the dream images into language only produces second-hand information concerning the actual, unobservable process'.[18] Thus drawing is the source of first-hand dream material while telling (or perhaps writing) moves further away into the second or third realm.

Bristol participant Toni, quoted above, made a special note of the difference between drawing and telling a dream and indicated her clear preference for drawing. From her perspective, drawing a dream can 'capture it in a way that writing can't … There's not often a word for what I have in dreams'. She explained: 'It does something that writing can't do'. Another interviewee noted: 'The picture always reminds you of the fact that you can't express everything in words'.

Combining verbal and drawing

Stefan Hau, whose research on dream drawing at the Freud Institute in Frankfurt was a critical resource for my doctoral work, advises that both the verbal telling and the picture are necessary. Although he demonstrates in his research the great advantages of drawing dreams, he notes that a drawing often does not allow for the narrative of a dream in action that a verbal retelling offers. Not only are dreams visual, but they are also ongoing in time and movement and not easy to capture visually; drawing can only capture a moment in a dream or a series of moments in a series of successive pictures.

In order for the contents of the dream to be understood or at least related to, it needs to be accompanied by a verbal description of the dream and some orientation to the images in the drawing. Otherwise, the observer cannot really make much of the meaning of the drawing. From Hau's perspective, the two modes complement and support one another. The combination of 'picture information' and 'text information'[19] provides a fuller and more whole 'picture' of the dream.

Other advantages in drawing dreams ...

As to the power and significance of drawing in general, it is interesting to remind ourselves of a very popular saying, 'A picture is worth a thousand words'. Even the simplest drawing can be very, very complex in that it has the potential to contain so much meaning and information. Unlike a verbal exposition, it does not just stand in for a single concept, nor is it a form of linear expression. In one view, you can see the entire Gestalt of the dream. Every point relates to the other points in the drawing. Even without intending, the drawing represents the unconscious processes in the dreamer from which much can be made in the free association process.

Taking the time to draw an important dream also has the advantage of slowing down the process of recreating and recalling the dream. In contrast to the speed with which we can talk, drawing a dream involves a series of decisions (where to draw, on what, with what) and launches one on the complicated process of recalling the dream images and then reconstructing them somehow. In the very first group I worked with, which met in Haarlem and Amsterdam, one participant described to me in detail all of the effort she took to find the right place (a cosy chair), time (after her son was in bed) and materials (her son's crayons) to capture her dreams (and, yes, the figure of her son did appear in some of her dreams). All of this allows for a deep inner process of remembering and sensing the original dream experience.

One can also argue that because we are so comfortable with talking and with telling our stories and experiences in our own words – often with elaborations or exaggerations that suit an entertaining narrative – we can tell others our dreams the way we want them to be told. We can easily make up our own version of reality or dream-ality, even relating a dream and particular elements of it to fit into an existing idea or self-narrative.

But with drawings, this sort of camouflage is not so easy. When one conceives of pictures as 'direct communications from the unconscious', as Furth does,[20] then unconscious meanings and feelings can be discerned. Sometimes it is how a person is drawn (with or without features, for example), or how strongly lines are drawn, or which colours predominate and where on the page they appear, etc. Of course, when one draws, one is conscious and one has an idea or a series of ideas as one tries to capture both the images of the inner eye and its narratives; but drawings in general, as Sapochnik notes, make unconscious material more available by 'circumventing internal censorship'.[21] Especially when the drawer allows others to offer their associations to the drawings, these freely drawn figures and styles come more and more to awareness and provide fascinating new material to consider during a difficult transitional time.

Perhaps this is best illustrated by the example of the missing red cross in the verbal retelling of a dream that surprisingly appeared in the dream drawing itself.

In every Social Dream-Drawing workshop, we work for one hour with each dream drawing. Before the dream drawer actually shows the drawing, she describes the dream to the group (so that group members can form their own mental pictures of the dream). Then the dreamer shows them her dream drawing, which she has brought from home.

One dream drawer in the Chilean group, having first spoken about his dream and then having shown the drawing to the group, realised with shock that when he verbally relayed his dream, he had forgotten a key symbolic element that appeared in the picture (see Figure 2.1). This element was a red cross drawn on the sheet covering the sick man (himself) in the hospital. It was the only colour in the entire drawing.

During the group's associations to this drawing, it became quite clear that the red cross symbolised not just the well-known international charity organisation. Instead, it stood for the role of the Catholic Church in Chile and had a direct connection to the issue the dream was addressing, i.e. the ability of this participant to support his family and be self-employed. Thus the missing red cross in the verbal telling of the dream that surprisingly appeared in the drawing turned out to be a key element in the meaning and message of the dream.

In this case, one could further hypothesise that the red cross, omitted in the telling of the dream, represented a particular danger that the dreamer

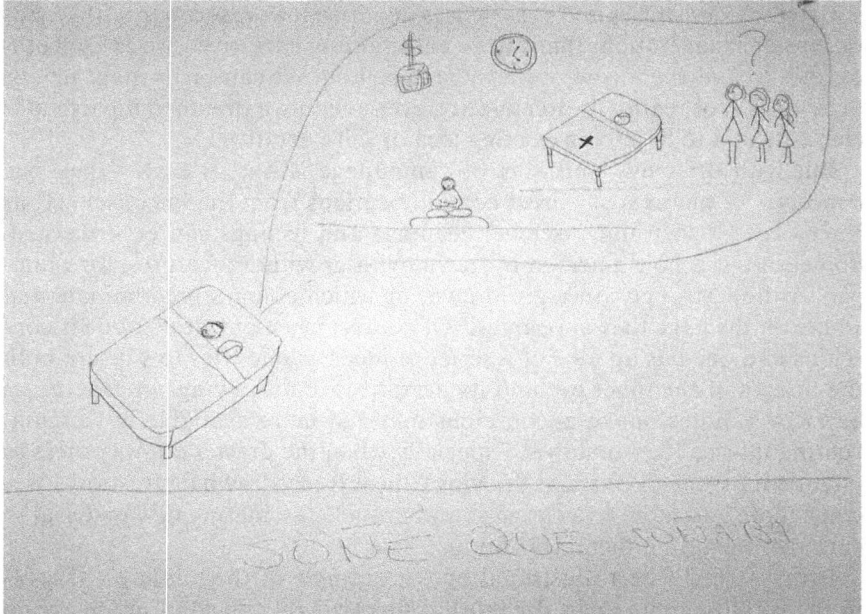

Figure 2.1 The red cross on the bed sheet

had already repressed by the time he came to the workshop. It was one of the participants who pointed it out.

One last critical advantage of drawing dreams is its value when working across international boundaries. As Taylor points out, images 'transcend the barriers of different languages and enhance communication in an increasingly global world'.[22] This has a great advantage for those from different cultures and countries, who belong to the same Social Dream-Drawing workshop. Typical situations would be those being moved by their employer from one country to another, or those doing a PhD at a foreign university. In these situations, the drawn dream serves as a bridge between cultures. My own research and further workshops, which were conducted with groups in six different countries, confirm this advantage.

The challenges of drawing a dream

When you think about it, it makes a lot of sense to draw one's dreams. After all, dreams are essentially visual. When we dream, we see images. We see events taking place. Sometimes we see ourselves. Sometimes we see people we have long forgotten. Often we see our parents and our loved ones. But essentially, we see.

However, it is really not so easy to draw a dream.

As we well know, dream images are often chaotic, confusing and impossible to describe, much less draw. After all, the dream drawer is not sketching from a model before her, nor is she painting something she has actually seen. The drawing is not an imitation and is not designed as a reproduction.

In technical terms, it is the associative cortex (one part of the visual cortex in our brains) that retrieves visual memories from the day and transforms them into dream material. In that sense, dream images are picture metaphors of associated memories, concepts and feelings and quite difficult to capture. Even though, as one of the participants in the London research group put it: 'Our mind recreates the external world'. Yes, but in such chaotic ways!

German researcher Hau calls the process of drawing a dream – the memory and the synthesis required, the transformation and the manufacturing challenges and skills needed – an 'extremely complex self-achievement'.[23] In the drawing process, the drawer has revisited the dream experience, which demands a great deal of energy, self-investment and 'psychic energy'.[24]

Artist Angela Eames emphasises that much effort is necessary in the 'search to produce some form of physical equivalence to the ideas swirling around in his head',[25] which is certainly not easy. And in drawing dreams, one is always aware of how quickly these fleeting images can disappear. So the act of drawing is a way 'to put down an idea before it floats away – to materialize an idea'.[26]

Another way to think about drawing dreams, however, is not so much to copy this unique image (or set of images), but instead to recapture the meaningfulness of the dream experience itself in such a way as to make it recognisable to others.[27] In this sense, it is really more a process of interpretation than of recall and representation. As such, one can say that drawing is an essential way of accessing this one-off, original and meaningful dream material. As Christine, my German research participant, noted in her interview: 'Drawing brings the inside out'.

In addition to the challenges of revisiting the original dream and of then capturing the images on paper, the dream drawer faces the problem of capturing a series of dream images in one drawing. A German newspaper article describes the experience of dreaming as *nächtliche Kopfkino* (nightly head cinema). This requires 'translating' a three-dimensional experience into a two-dimensional medium.[28] This might be considered comparable to being asked to draw a movie or a television series on one piece of paper. How and what do you choose?

The dreamers in my study found many creative ways to handle this. Heike, in the German research group, used two different ways of drawing her dreams in multiple images (see Figure 2.2a and b). Figure 2.2a involved a dream about opening an apple and discovering something rotten inside. The steps in this process were drawn from the top to the bottom of the page.

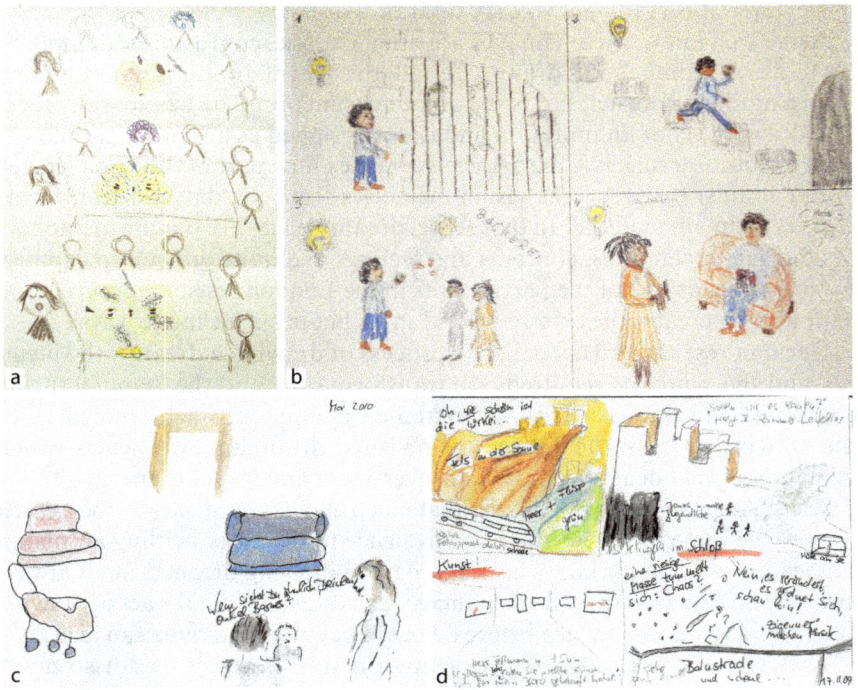

Figure 2.2 Capturing dreams on paper

Figure 2.2b is organised in four quadrants. In this complex dream, Heike escorts a lost little boy through a tunnel into a bakery. Christine, also in the German research group, drew two contrasting examples (see Figure 2.2c and d). In Figure 2.2c, she captures a few fragments from a dream, particularly pieces of furniture. In Figure 2.2d, she drew four different dreams on one piece of paper, each with its own special images.

For those participating in Social Dream-Drawing workshops, probably the greatest challenge to drawing a dream is the stress level of the person drawing it. Many participants feel insecure about drawing in general and representing dream material specifically. Many feel they are not talented enough for this feat. Some feel ashamed to do something so childish and to share it with others. Since these drawings will be brought into a group, they often experience a form of performance anxiety related to judgements and interpretations of their creations. Attempts to compensate for a perceived lack of talent can bring the drawing even further away from the dream material. And the really talented drawers can sometimes over-perform in creating lovely-to-look at drawings.

The advantages of drawing dreams

There are many advantages to drawing one's dreams. Drawings can capture the intrinsic visual nature of dreams and allow a richer and broader world of unconscious meanings to emerge. Drawing a dream slows down the process of remembering and brings the dreamer back to the same sort of regressive frame of mind as experienced when dreaming.

Very often, important details emerge in the drawings that are not present in the linear and logical sequence of verbalisation. On the other hand, the act of transporting a unique inner visual image into a two-dimensional form is certainly not easy and poses a definite limitation to this method. When dreams are shared using both mediums (verbal and pictorial), a space for the integration of unconscious elements with conscious thinking opens up to create deep learning opportunities.

All in all, without a dream drawing, this deep experience just stays inside of us. A colourful, expressive drawing brings it out of us and makes it available to others!

Notes

1 Freud, S. (1900) *The Interpretation of Dreams.* S.E. Volume 4-5. Reprint. Middlesex: Penguin, 1976.
2 See Hau (2004, pp. 91–8), for an extensive elaboration.
3 Jung, C.G. (1930) *The Red Book: Liber Novus.* Reprint. New York: The Philemon Foundation & W.W. Norton & Co., 2009.
4 Shafton, A. (1995) *Dream Reader: Contemporary Approaches to the Understanding of Dreams.* Albany, NY: SUNY Press, p. 383.

5 Fay, B. (2013) *What Is Drawing – A Continuous Incompleteness*. Dublin: Irish Museum of Modern Art, p. 16.
6 Van Alphen, E. (2012) Looking at drawing: theoretical distinctions and their usefulness. In: Garner, S., ed., *Writing on Drawing: Essays on Drawing Practice and Research*. Bristol: Intellect, p. 62.
7 Hau, S. (2004) *Träume zeichnen: Über die visuelle Darstellung von Traumbildern*. Tübingen: edition discord.
8 Ibid., p. 109.
9 Ibid., p. 201.
10 Sapochnik, C. (2013) Drawing below the surface: eliciting tacit knowledge in social science research. *Tracey*. Special Edition developed from selected papers at the 2012 Doctoral Research Conference (DRC) at Loughborough University, p. 13.
11 Fischer, C. (1957) A study of the preliminary stages of the constructions of dreams and images. *Journal of the American Psychoanalytic Association*. 5, p. 36.
12 Arnheim, R. (1969) *Visual Thinking*. Berkeley: University of California Press, p. 244.
13 Ibid.
14 Ibid.
15 Ibid., p. 245.
16 Ibid., p. 246.
17 Langer, S. (1960) *Philosophy in a New Key*. Cambridge: Harvard University Press, p. 65.
18 Walde, C. (1999) Dream interpretation in a prosperous age? In: Shulman, D. & Stroumsa, G.G., eds., *Dream Cultures: Explorations in the Comparative History of Dreaming*. New York: Oxford University Press, p. 131.
19 Hau, S. (2004) *Träume zeichnen: Über die visuelle Darstellung von Traumbildern*. Tübingen: edition discord, p. 111.
20 Furth, G.M. (1988) *The Secret World of Drawings – Healing Through Art*. Boston, MA: Sigo Press, p. 4.
21 Sapochnik, C. (2012) The use of drawing as a research tool in social research [lecture to UWE postgraduate psycho-social group seminar]. University of West England, Bristol, UK. 14 November.
22 Taylor, A. (2012) Forward – re: positioning drawing. In: Garner, S., ed., *Writing on Drawing: Essays on Drawing Practice and Research*. Bristol: Intellect, p. 10.
23 Hau, S. (2004) *Träume zeichnen: Über die visuelle Darstellung von Traumbildern*. Tübingen: edition discord, p. 202.
24 Ibid., p. 208.
25 Eames, A. (2012) Embedded drawing. In: Garner, S., ed., *Writing on Drawing: Essays on Drawing Practice and Research*. Bristol: Intellect, p. 35.
26 Ibid., p. 127.
27 Hau, S. (2004) *Träume zeichnen: Über die visuelle Darstellung von Traumbildern*. Tübingen: edition discord, p. 119.
28 Ibid., p. 141.

Chapter 3

The support and learning from group work

Let's face it, groups are not easy. They are not for everyone. As the British analyst Wilfred Bion pointed out in his 1961 classic book, *Experiences in Groups and Other Papers*,[1] being in a group can threaten our individual identity. We are not sure if we will survive.

This can be especially so in a group exploring dream material. Here, we do not have the familiarity of a problem to solve or an agenda to fulfil. We don't know what to expect, how we will feel, or whether the effort will even be worth it.

Contemporary research demonstrates that in many difficult life situations, such as coping with loneliness, caring for a relative at home or finishing a PhD, participating in groups of like-minded people has a healing and motivating effect. Malcolm Pines, a British group analyst, emphasises 'the transformational potential of the group situation'.[2] He describes group analytic work similarly to Social Dream-Drawing (SDD), in that it is based on 'the understanding that people meet together in order to increase their understanding of themselves and thereby to gain greater mastery over their inner lives'.[3] SDD has at its core the assumption that work with dream drawings can be greatly enhanced by a group of people who are going through the same transitional experience.

I found this to be true, for example, with a group of doctoral students in London in a workshop that formed part of my research. Three of the four participants were going through the same doctoral programme, and all three brought dream drawings relating to earlier professional roles (and role dilemmas), which resurfaced as they, once more, started over as students. One role pattern that emerged was that of belonging nowhere, and many of the visual images were of leaving or not recognising houses. This is a common visual theme in SDD.

Why is it, then, that sharing dream drawings in a group is so valuable?

At the most practical level, group work means that all may benefit from the ideas and resources of others. You are likely to come into contact with people who have already explored the problematic issue at hand and who have developed particular strategies or found some good resources for coping with it. Simply exchanging this sort of information is already a bonus.

DOI: 10.4324/9780429275647-4

As a member of a group, you are obliged to talk and communicate: *Why I am here? What I am looking for? Who I am?* Communicating this information, in and of itself, helps each member articulate where he is and what he needs in his life. That is often the first step towards a deeper understanding of a situation.

Group participation reduces the sense of isolation. In a group, you very soon realise you are not the only one dealing with a particular problem or situation. That alone is helpful. In fact, one could say that group contact, even without particular resources or problem formulation, can have a healing and helpful effect. You are lifted out of your personal inner state of mind and into a social context. It can be a relief to hear others discuss what they're going through, and to realise you're not alone.

This turned out to be especially so for the online group that I ran (see Chapter 9), when there was no possibility of in-person social follow-up. One participant later commented that, as difficult as it was to be confronted with the dream drawings and the issues they raised, this forum was the only one she had where she could truly share her deeper experiences of the virus. It was, for her, a safe and open space, where she could deeply experience the terror and sadness she experienced. In all other areas of her life, like the rest of us, she just had to get on with it.

In a well-facilitated group, participation promotes self-esteem. As a member, you are valuable, and you will be valuable to everyone in this group. Others are in need as well, and you can help them. The experience of offering emotional support to others, even at a time of personal crisis, increases a sense of worth. This creates hope.

Here is how London participant Frederick described his experience:

> There was a real eureka moment, really, and I certainly enjoyed talking about my dreams. They're something so intimate that we kind of keep to ourselves and when you put it out there to see what other people make of it, also helps you think about it yourself really. It's a very enjoyable experience in terms of sharing and hearing other peoples' as well, actually .... I think when you're showing it to other people you see it again yourself .... And I think see it through other peoples' eyes really struck home and made very, very powerful ... I thought, 'My God, this is very powerful.' And it felt both exposing and exciting at the same time. That was the moment I felt I was on a cliff edge in the group as well; it felt quite risky and the adrenaline was flowing.

Very often, the benefits of this work take time to be integrated. In my interview with Fran, a member of the London research group, she realised, after some time had passed, what the work had meant to her. Here is how she expressed it:

> ... there's a transition I'm going through professionally which is about being much clearer about the limits of what I can do if the resources

aren't there ... I have a kind of heroic tendency to soldier on come hell or high water ... I'm [now] at [the] stage where if something can't be done, it can't be done ... So some of what I was revisiting in my dreams were some very long struggles with some very difficult people and actually knowing what I know now, I should have just walked away from them on day two! (*Laughs*.) Rather than on day one hundred and two or whatever and by then you're in and it's not so easy to get out ... [I]f you've been struggling on heroically and you're depleting your own resources, you're not in a good place at that point to negotiate.

So I think that the experience of being part of your group and working with you and working with colleagues has helped me get a bit more in touch with the sort of professional that I want to be at this point in my life and my professional journey.

Bringing social dreams to the group

In addition to the basic benefits of group work, as outlined above, working specifically on drawings of dreams in a group context generates rich and deep data for constructive exploration and intensive insight.

Why is that so?

To begin with, there is the notion that there is an ongoing connection between the waking self and the sleeping self, in the sense that our conscious thoughts have a continuous connection with those of our dreams. As such, as the contemporary psychoanalyst Christopher Bollas puts it, 'the night self begins *knowingly* to dream *for* the day self'.[4] And from Bollas's perspective, this allows the two parts to work in 'partnership'.[5] As one German participant put it, the SDD experience 'brings together what was separated, i.e. the conscious with the unconscious, the individual with the group'.

SDD is partly based on the notion that dreams themselves are produced in relation to a specific context, meaning in direct connection to a situation or relationship in one's daily life. Psychotherapists like to joke that patients dream particular dreams in order to bring them as gifts to their therapists. I think that is so. The dream and the dream drawing that the Wolf Man offered to Freud is a good example of that (see Chapter 2). So in SDD, by having a particular animating theme, participants bring those dream drawings that are relevant to this question for the group to work on.

In developing Social Dreaming, from which SDD evolved, Gordon Lawrence based his methodology on Jung's concept that there are different kinds of dreams.[6] Jung differentiated personal dreams, dealing with the daily lives of dreamers, from what he called dreams from the collective unconscious. For Jung, 'Personal dreams are limited to the affairs of everyday life and one's personal process, offering information and guidance pertaining to what is going on in our current lives. These are the everyday dreams, the "bread and butter" of the dream world'.[7] The collective dreams have a much broader meaning. Thus they are more appropriate for group work with dreams and dream drawings.

Lawrence posited that the context of Social Dreaming leads participants to 'produce' social dreams. From his perspective, the dreamer (or more specifically, the dreamer's unconscious) knows what it is doing, as my own work has confirmed. The key concept here is that the individual dreams on behalf of the group, in the sense that, when worked on collectively, the dream offers insights into a theme or an issue that all participants share, such as 'What do I risk in my transition?' or 'Who am I online?'

What is the difference between a personal dream and a social dream?

One way of answering that is to consider to whom the dream actually belongs. Personal dreams are those a patient brings to a therapeutic session and are 'properly regarded as possessions of the dreamer ... that foster the therapeutic process'.[8] This would include dreams about one's childhood and family figures, personal relationships and even sexual encounters, for example.

Social dreams are those dreams relating to concerns of the social world. They can include world events, professional or work-related issues, relocation, and social upheavals. They contain dream material relating to the social world.

Participants are asked to bring whatever dream drawing they wish to SDD. Sometimes a personal dream is presented, but mostly participants bring social dreams. Dreamers control what they bring and what they want to work on. Because the participant knows in advance that whatever dream drawing he or she brings will be worked on in the group, it is more likely that the nature of the dream material itself will be primarily of a social nature, as opposed to a highly personal dream.

Each workshop or set of workshops has a particular theme, which is based on the particular transition being experienced by participants. I like to word all the themes in the form of a question, because this type of phrasing invites consideration and suggests there may be multiple influences on a particular transition. I base the themes on issues typical for this group. For example, for doctoral students, I have used topics such as: 'Who am I as researcher?' For new organisational consultants, a profession involving great uncertainty about being self-employed, I have used the theme: 'What do I risk in my work?' For a multi-generation graduate research course, I have used: 'How does my generation influence my research?'

Only dreams and dream drawings taking place after the theme is announced are allowed to be worked on in the group. Participants are encouraged to draw many dreams and then choose one to bring to the group. This increases the chance that their dream drawings will relate directly to the theme. For example, a dream relating to a work conflict would be more likely to be shared than one regarding sexual relations, even though both dreams may be highly significant to the individual. Giving participants control over which drawing to bring creates a sense of safety, as dream material is often quite personal. About six weeks before the first workshop, I send out a detailed letter explaining the method and advising participants on how to remember their dreams, or as one colleague put it, how to 'train their dream-capturing muscle'.

How working on dream drawings fosters cohesion and connection

In the previous chapter on the drawing of dreams, I discussed the way in which the drawing creates a bridge between the inner world of the dreamer and his conscious self. This two-dimensional representation of the dream functions physically as a link between the dreamer and the original dream material.

This metaphor of a bridge can be applied to the group experience as well. The deep focus on each dream drawing enables group members to connect to the dreamer's inner dream material and therefore to the dreamer's inner world. Thus one can say that the drawing lives in two worlds: the world of the dreamer and the world of the group undertaking its task.

Because the drawing is a separate object, it brings distance and perspective. In addition, it functions as a form of safety net for the dreamer, in that the attention of the group goes to the drawing and not to the unconscious of the dreamer personally. Paradoxically, at the same time, as a linking object, it fosters integration. It connects something originating in the unconscious to the larger world.

When the dream is thought about as a separate object in this way, the dreamer can also experience a different kind of perspective on her original dream. Because of this, the dreamer is actually able to associate to her drawing in the course of the workshop. As such, the original dream material is reactivated, which sometimes evokes previously unremembered original fragments. These are then shared with the group. One vivid example of this phenomenon was described in the previous chapter, relating to the man in Chile who originally left out the red cross symbolising the Catholic Church when describing his dream.

In terms of psychoanalytic theory, there are different ways of thinking about the dream drawing. Feminist psychoanalyst Jessica Benjamin uses the term 'shared third'[9] to describe what is created between patient and analyst during the course of treatment. It is a shared reality and experience that exists between them yet outside of each of them as individuals. In the work of SDD, it is the drawing that serves this function. It is physically separate, yet when used in the work, it forms the basis of a shared working experience that all can relate to and extract meaning from.

With respect to the way in which a group works with dream drawings, there is often a very playful aspect. The notion of play in group work comes from the British child analyst Donald Winnicott.[10] He was fascinated with the role of play in childhood development. For him, children's play was somehow a kind of rehearsal for adult life. In playing, the child could, in a risk-free environment, repeatedly rehearse and conquer the challenges posed by the external world, including that of separating from the mother. In this 'potential' or 'transitional' play space, the child gradually discovers and develops its sense of identity.

In this process of separation and identity development, external objects, such as a teddy bear, stand in for the mother when the two are separated. Winnicott's term for such things is a 'transitional object', coined in his 1971 book *Playing and Reality*.[11] Through the use of, and interaction with, various objects, which he saw as symbolising the mother from whom he or she was gradually separating, the child would transition into an independent and self-confident person. When this approach is applied to SDD, the drawing functions similarly as a transitional object.

And just as a child's teddy bear becomes a treasured object to the child, the dream drawing itself often functions the same way. It is a physical reminder of a group experience that was transformational and which supported the participant at a time of great upheaval in his or her life. In bringing the deeply personal out and shared safely with others, it stands for an experience of great emotional meaning.

How does the group work with the dream drawings?

In some ways, it is easier to say what we do not do when working on the drawings. We do not attempt to analyse the symbolic significance of the images (e.g. that a dream drawing of someone falling relates to anxieties about letting go, losing control or somehow failing after a success). Additionally, we do not use the dream material to interpret or analyse the dreamer, which is usually the source of most peoples' anxiety about sharing their dreams. And we do not interpret their general meaning (e.g. 'this is a dream about the loss of people we love') or make deductions from them about the dreamers (e.g. 'this person must be very unhappy').

Instead, we use what is before us and what we have just heard from the dreamer as a springboard for sharing our own inner thoughts. This process, touched upon earlier, is called free association (*freie assoziation*) and is a method of inquiry developed by Sigmund Freud.[12] When one free associates, one says whatever comes to mind in as uncensored way as possible. In SDD, this means that all participants say whatever comes to mind in relation to the dream drawing they are focusing on.

Free associations come in countless forms.

Sometimes it has to do with the colours in the drawing (e.g. 'lots of blue intersecting black lines'). Sometimes a drawn item reminds one of an animal (for example, 'I can see an octopus') or a person ('Ronald Reagan') one is familiar with. Sometimes it has to do with how the drawing itself is set on the paper ('the page is completely full, there's no free space left on it!').

A dream drawing may call to mind earlier personal experiences ('I'm thinking of my child's accident when horse riding') or even one's recent dream ('my father living in a big brown warehouse ...').

Free associations can also be in the form of amplifications, a concept developed by C.J. Jung.[13] Amplifications are those cultural and political elements that come to mind, such as current events, music, literature and film. Thus one might refer to a recent exhibition at the Tate Modern ('the lines in this drawing remind me of the artwork where there was a line gashed in the floor') or a recent public event ('I see Meghan and Prince Harry's wedding night!').

During this process, it is not necessary for these associations to make sense and they are often very funny. One sees all sorts of things in a dream drawing, and we do have a good time playing with them in these workshops. Nevertheless, work is being done, what South African neuropsychologist Mark Solms[14] calls 'serious play' and 'playing for real'.

What is the point of this? Why free association?

Free association may seem pointless, but it has a very important purpose. Although, when free associating, it might appear that people are moving from one topic to another in a random way, there is actually an associative thought process going on within the group as a whole. One person's association stimulates another person's. One person's free and playful association leads to others. In the freewheeling and often fun experience of free association, 'a chain of ideas'[15] begins to form. These chains of ideas are often in the form of recurring themes that are later explored.

However, at this stage of the process, the nature of these ideas and what they mean are not the focus. Participants are simply free to react and comment. In and of itself, this brings the group into a mutual experience of creativity, fun and play, which is valuable in bringing about a sense of connection. The dream drawer and the facilitator actively participate as well, which encourages a sense of joint fun.

It is worth noting that free association does not come easily to everyone. It can take time to become comfortable offering up what may seem completely strange thoughts. It is especially not so easy to do in a group, because participants realise that they may be inadvertently revealing something about themselves. Comments they might normally keep to themselves sometimes stay that way, and every participant is perfectly free to draw that boundary for themselves. That said, there are times when people make associations that in some way hurt the dreamer (e.g. 'there is too much detail in this drawing. I can't work with it!'). In these circumstances, i.e. when fun tilts a bit too far into shame or criticism, it is the role of the facilitator to make space for this experience to be discussed and hopefully clarified. (see Chapter 8 on Facilitation Skills).

For some participants, it is never possible to get beyond what is on the page ('it's an aeroplane' or 'I like the colours'). Learning to free associate and feeling comfortable in a group takes time and practice. One must first feel safe and not subject to scrutiny or judgement. Sometimes sexual associations make people uncomfortable. The facilitator seeks to contain this concern by not censoring or criticising, and by sometimes offering the occasional risky association of her own. One example I remember clearly was an association I made to a dream drawing, which, from my perspective, was upside down. To me it looked like an octopus. At first, this association shocked the group, but they soon realised that, depending on one's perspective, anything is possible. In the process, group members learn together. Gradually they experience a sense of safety and acceptance and start to enjoy the experience. So sometimes, the facilitator has to look the fool before others will join in!

After the 15-minute free association phase, the dreamer is given the opportunity to respond. Although it is often tempting for the dreamer to comment or clarify on the dream drawing during the free association period, I encourage them to allow the flow of associations, since they will later have their turn to comment. Very often, the dreamers are truly amazed by what group members have 'seen' in their drawings. Some free associations, while seemingly random to group members, often seem to be spot on to the dreamer. As one of my research participants put it:

> I am so amazed at your associations. It never occurred to me that these small huts that I drew were all actually connected to different parts of me (i.e. the small broken-down hut and the nicely decorated hut). Yes, that's me! Thank you so much!

After the dreamer responds, the group work continues in a new direction with a 20-minute reflection phase. The group's new task is to try to understand the themes expressed in the free associations and to explore their links with the theme of the workshop. In order to take on this task, the participants must be helped to emerge from the regressive state of free association and enter the more familiar state of group discussion and reflection. At the suggestion of my doctoral supervisor, I incorporate a bit of physical movement into the workshop at this stage, in order to help participants return to their bodies and thus become more reintegrated with a normal group experience. I ask every one (including myself) to stand up and move to another person's seat. For online groups, I ask participants to stand up and take a small walk around their apartment or work space. This small physical exercise marks an important transition in task and state.

In the 20-minute reflection period, participants are asked to try to make some sense of the free association phase. They are asked to do this in different ways. One way is by identifying patterns in the associations, e.g. 'Gosh, there were a lot of associations about wild animals, weren't there?' Another way is to recall an especially intense emotion experienced during the association phase, e.g. 'I couldn't believe how angry I got at this drawing'. The dreamer is especially encouraged to comment, e.g. 'I didn't realise how many times I failed to draw the features on the faces'.

In order to maximise the practicality of this phase, the facilitator reminds the group of the theme of the workshop, and participants are also encouraged to think about this. As we have seen, the themes can include broad questions such as the following: 'What do I risk in my work?' or 'Who am I as researcher?' or 'Where do I belong?' While it is not always so easy to make this jump from making free associations to analysing the themes, some are able to. Comments include: 'Sometimes I am afraid to fill up the page, like the dream drawing, when I interview for a new job. I only show them a small part of my page'. Or: 'The picture of the poisoned apple made me think of the poisonous colleagues in my consulting firm, one trying to eliminate the other'.

As referred to in Chapter 4, in the fall of 2020, I conducted an online workshop with ten participants. Four of them participated in the work on the dream drawing, while the other six observed the process. When it came to the phase of thinking about the theme, it was the observers who offered many good insights. This made me realise that SDD could work very well with larger groups. One group could work on the dream drawing and the observers could have the important role of reflecting on the theme. In the fall of 2021, with my colleague, Anton Zemlyanoy, I organised a further online dream drawing workshop, which made use of this idea of an observing group (see further discussion in Chapter 4).

It is fair to say that this is just the beginning of the learning experience for the participants. Things are not neatly wrapped up at the end of each workshop. Food for thought has only just begun, as they return to their regular lives. A deep process has been initiated that, over a period of time, begins to impact their transitional experience, whatever it may be. Over the course of a workshop, when participants have shared many dream drawings, patterns emerge and a certain kind of integration occurs. This has been made clear over and over again in the interviews I have conducted with participants.

For example, Frederick in the London group remarked that our work on his dream drawing (see Figure 3.1) made him aware of how separated he was from his own family, as his giant figure loomed over all that was going on in his life.

In reflecting on the drawing, he could see that while, on the one hand, he has 'long legs and roots firmly placed' and is 'somehow holding things together', he could also see the 'lack of communication with family' and a

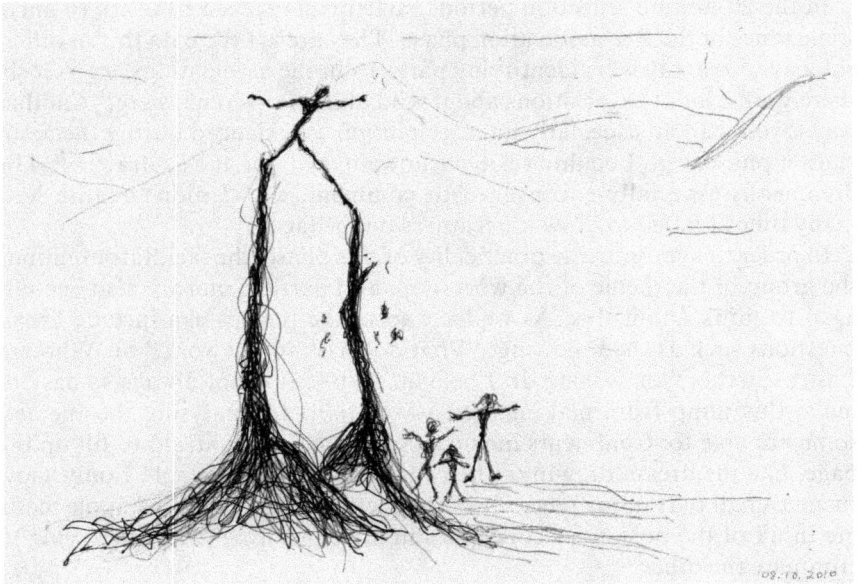

Figure 3.1 The tall man

general 'difficulty in making connections with others'. He began to realise the price he may be paying for his professional success and wondered if he truly had everything in control. As he said:

> Still higher to go .... could be my need to keep pushing never quite good enough – not even with a doctorate – what next!!!? Omnipotence before a fall? Or can confidence take you through?

He realised it was an important time of 'risk and opportunities'.

The rewards of free association and reflection

As stated above, there are many social and emotional benefits to working in a group, especially during a time of transition. Common issues are identified and mutual support increases. But the method of SDD provides participants with much more than this. Not only are their emotional and social needs supported, but participants also gain greater insight into the deeper issues they are personally experiencing in relation to their individual transitions. And these insights and learnings provide guidance and support in navigating these changes.

Sometimes an insight is relevant to the entire group, such as when a dream drawing applies to issues broader than the immediate concerns of the

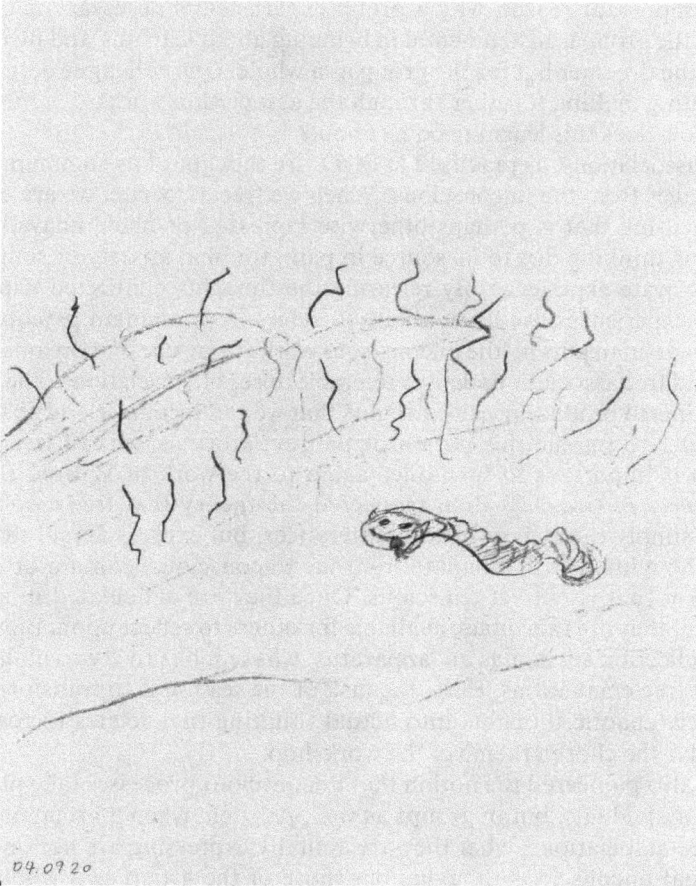

04.09.20

Figure 3.2 Coronavirus worm

dreamer him- or herself. One recent example is the dream drawing shown in Figure 3.2, which is by a participant in a group working with the theme 'What do I risk in my transition?'

In this dream, Tom is lying down on his back and looking at his stomach. Out of his stomach, little wiggling worms are coming up. One big red one is looking directly at him. Our associations to this dream drawing led to the idea that the red worm represents the coronavirus and the way in which it is preventing all of the participants from engaging in their transition into retirement. New interests cannot be pursued. New courses cannot be taken. We, just like the dreamer, are caught sleeping on our backs.

This was a great insight to this dreamer, whose own retirement plans had been severely limited by the virus.

One important reason why a group experience is necessary is that the work of the group is instrumental in bringing about learning and insight not just for the dreamer but for the group as a whole. One colleague described it as 'meaning making together through the association work'.

But how does this learning come about?

Free associations, as practised in SDD, are thought of as communications or messages from the unconscious. When we free associate, we are expressing something that is perhaps otherwise repressed or made unavailable to conscious thinking due to its source in pain, trauma, anxiety or some other deeply private experience. By releasing the thoughts connected with these difficult experiences, we learn about ourselves. As Canadian psychoanalyst Keith Haartman puts it: 'the unconscious works to ensure that dreams, symptoms, and free associations deliver tolerable doses of "revelation". The unconscious aims to produce useable insights that we can recognise and absorb'.[16]

In order to pursue this notion of the revelatory aspects of free association, it is important to turn once again to the work of Wilfred Bion. In *Experiences in Groups,*[17] Bion pioneered the theory that free associations are not simply random or chaotic utterances, but express actual thoughts. These thoughts, which emanate from the unconscious, contain or express a problem that is not yet conscious. Once they are articulated in a group situation, they are then made available for others to reflect upon. Bion refers to the reflection session as an 'apparatus' whose job is to try to make sense of these free emanations. Here, the task of the session is to transform these seemingly chaotic thoughts into actual thinking that relates to reality, in particular the chosen theme of the workshop.

Bion also pioneered the notion that unconscious processes take place not only in individuals, but in groups as well. As such, when a group of people offer free associations, what they are actually expressing are not only their individual unconscious thoughts but those of the group as a whole. Even when someone offers a wild statement, it can be seen as not just a thought from that individual, but from the group too. This increases the resources of the group as a whole, owing to the wisdom contained in the collective unconscious thoughts.

Marking a key transitional experience

As stated above, group experiences offer support and connection during times of transition. The work of the SDD group, in addition, leads to insights relating to the challenges of the transition in question. Another significant advantage of dream drawings is that they function as a permanent visual reminder of an important emotional group experience. Unlike told dreams, which are soon forgotten, or even written dreams which, when re-read, somehow lose their resonance, the dream drawing exists and persists in one's life long after the end of the workshop experience.

This phenomenon is confirmed by my own research. Bristol participant Toni noted that she can still remember the dream that she drew, as opposed to other dreams that she had at the same time that she didn't draw. She is able to 'recall the image in my mind very clearly'. In addition, the drawing 'brings back the emotion' associated with the original dream experience.

The long-term resonance of the visual is emphasised by University of Pennsylvania professor of communication Barbie Zelizer. As she notes: 'how we remember through images remains powerfully different from how we might remember the same event were images not involved'.[18] Here she explains how drawings stay in the memory over time and support our capacity to remember:

> As vehicles of memory, images work in patterned ways, concretizing and externalizing events in an accessible and visible fashion that allows us to recognize the tangible proof they offer of the events being represented. Images actively depend on their material form when operating as vehicles of memory, with our ability to remember events of the past facilitated by an image's availability and interchangeability. In a sense, then, visual memory's texture becomes a facilitator for memory's endurance.[19]

A dream drawing can be continually returned to. It can be displayed in your office or in a special album or diary. And because it has been worked on so deeply with a group, it stands not just for the original dream itself, but also for the emotional experience and insights that have arisen with the group.

As such, the dream drawing can be thought of as an important transitional object, like Winnicott's teddy bear. The infant's teddy bear serves as a symbolic representation of the mother–infant union. And this object stands in for the experience of being held by the mother. When the mother is not physically present, this transitional link keeps the infant close to her and to their joint experience symbolically. The dream drawing functions in a similar way.

Even after many years have passed, the dream drawing serves as an important triggering device for memories relating to a major transitional time in an individual's life. Quite often, when I ask people from an earlier workshop if I may interview them about their experience, they will tell me at first that they can't remember anything. But as soon as they see the picture again, the experience comes back, in full colour, as it were. They see the drawing again, and the experience is revived.

This significance can even take place when it is someone else's dream drawing. For example, when I contacted a former participant who worked with the dream drawing of someone he was supervising, and asked him if he perhaps still had the original drawing, he replied:

> I DO REMEMBER! But I don't have the picture seven years ago. I can remember it etched in my mind like a flame – I could probably draw it but not like the original which was so, so powerful.

Why does the dream drawing manage to take on such a major role?

As mentioned, the dream drawing functions as a bridge between internal experience and objective reality. It brings these elements together in an integrative way, which is the process of working through a difficult transition. But it also brings together the members of the group. As one of my German participants put it: the drawing 'brings together what was separated, i.e. the conscious with the unconscious, the individual with the group'. It functions as a binding element in the group experience.

Thus, even when the original dream material may fade, the deep process of transition at that time in one's life stays alive. The drawing itself symbolises this process. As such, it functions as a mnemonic device (referred to in German as an *Eselsbrücke*), something that triggers important memories. This is certainly confirmed by the interviews I have done with participants, sometimes as much as three years later. For so many of them, the drawing acts as a symbol and souvenir of an important transitional time in their lives. And the group experience intensifies this memory and this transition.

Now that we have looked at the various theories underlying the practice of SDD, it is time to focus on the practicalities of running a workshop, including careful preparation, design, facilitation skills and ethics.

Notes

1 Bion, W.R. (1961) *Experiences in Groups and Other Papers*. London: Tavistock Publications.
2 Pines, M. (1994) The group-as-a-whole. In: Brown, D. & Zinken, L., eds., *Developments in Group-Analytic Theory*. London: Routledge, p. 52.
3 Ibid., p. 55.
4 Bollas, C. (2011) *The Christopher Bollas Reader*. London: Routledge, 254.
5 Ibid.
6 Lawrence, W.G. (2003) Social dreaming as sustained thinking. *Human Relations*. 56 (5), pp. 609–624.
7 Jung, C.G. (1930) *The Red Book: Liber Novus*. Reprint. New York: The Philemon Foundation & W.W. Norton & Co., 2009, p. 10.
8 Lawrence, W.G. (2003) Social dreaming as sustained thinking. *Human Relations*. 56 (5), p. 619.
9 Benjamin, J. (2004) Beyond doer and done to: an intersubjective view of thirdness. *Psychoanalytic Quarterly*. 73, p, 19.
10 Winnicott, D.W. (1971) *Playing and Reality*. Reprint. London: Routledge, 1996.
11 Ibid.
12 Freud, S. (1900) *The Interpretation of Dreams*. S.E. Volume 4-5. Reprint. Middlesex: Penguin, 1976.
13 Jung, C.G. (1961) *Memories, Dreams, Reflections*. Reprint. London: Fontana, 1995.
14 Solms, M. (2014) *Brain mechanisms underpinning some social processes*. [plenary presentation at annual conference of the Organisation for Promoting Understanding of Society (OPUS)] London, UK. 22 November.

15 Bollas, C. (2007) *The Freudian Moment: Second Edition*. Reprint. London: Karnac, 2013, p. 9.
16 Haartman, K. (no date) *Review of Grotstein, James S. (2000). Who Is the Dreamer Who Dreams the Dream?* Hillsdale: The Analytic Press. *Kleinian Studies Ejournal*. http://www.psychoanalysis-and-therapy.com/human_nature/ksej/hartmangrotstein.html. [accessed 08.09.2014].
17 Bion, W.R. (1961) *Experiences in Groups and Other Papers*. London: Tavistock Publications.
18 Zelizer, B (2004) The voice of the visual in memory. In: Phillips, K., ed., *Framing Public Memory*. Tuscaloosa: The University of Alabama Press, p. 158.
19 Ibid., p. 60.

Chapter 4

Organising and undertaking a Social Dream-Drawing workshop

As with putting on any major event, setting the stage and offering a welcoming and safe atmosphere is very important. Since Social Dream-Drawing (SDD) will be something completely foreign and perhaps a bit scary for most participants, I have devoted this chapter to the practicalities of hosting an SDD workshop.

In the pages that follow, I will be describing the preparatory steps for organising an SDD workshop, starting with the key question of why we would offer one in the first place. I will then discuss a number of issues relating to undertaking these sorts of workshops. They include: identifying a theme, assembling a group, rules for confidentiality and finding an appropriate venue. I will offer advice on the number of workshops to offer, how far apart they should be held and the question of whether dream drawings should be brought to the workshop or drawn in the workshop.

Why offer Social Dream-Drawing in the first place?

When considering whether to offer an SDD workshop, many different factors can come into play. We first have to be convinced that bringing a group into close contact with unconscious material that relates to current changes in their lives will really be beneficial to them. How do we make that judgement?

One key factor is how secure the facilitator feels in holding the workshop. As is thoroughly explained in Chapter 8, there are many factors that go into facilitating these workshops successfully. The facilitator himself must have certain skills that will allow for safe work and the containment of the sort of anxieties that are inherent in working with dream material.

It may, therefore, be best to start with a group of people who already have worked with dream material and/or who are interested in creative learning and growing experiences. In my case, I started off working with colleagues and former students who were familiar with a related method, Social Dreaming, and who were comfortable working with unconscious processes in groups.

DOI: 10.4324/9780429275647-5

It is important to emphasise that SDD is not, however, a therapeutic group experience, although it can have a therapeutic impact, in that it helps people better understand and work through personal anxieties. This means that participants who have been in group therapy may not easily adapt to the structure of SDD and the rules inherent in it. They may also not fully understand that the focus is on the drawing and not on the individual and his or her personal emotional history.

SDD can be particularly valuable when you are working with the same group over an extended period of time. It can supplement other training and professional development courses. It builds connections and lasting relationships. It can be offered as one option among a number of others by an institute or a university.

If we think of SDD as an intervention, then other factors come into play. Perhaps you have been working for a period of time with a number of nurses or accountants who are struggling to cope with group conflict or the unrelenting pressure of deadlines. Here, there is a direct problem in their working lives that has not heretofore been resolved by using more traditional group techniques. It is possible, under such circumstances, to propose an SDD workshop. A theme relating directly to the presenting issue could be developed with the group (for example, for the nurses, 'Who is healing the healer?' or for the accountants, 'Who is accounting for the accountant?'). And if this one-time experience proves valuable, then more workshops could be organised.

It is also worth noting that offering a one-off workshop to any set of participants, with the option to continue, is a very good way of getting direct feedback and helping a group decide whether to continue with the work. If offering multiple workshops, it is necessary for participants to commit to attending all the sessions (which is not always so easy). If people are forced to make this commitment and the first workshop is not experienced as particularly helpful, then one runs the risk of reduced numbers, which will affect the dynamics in the group.

Choosing a theme for the workshop

One of the cardinal principles of an SDD workshop is to identify a theme that relates directly to the challenges and anxieties around the changes that the participants are going through.

Although we talk about dreams as being purely unconscious and not influenced by our normal rational way of thinking, in fact, dreams always emerge from the context of the struggles in our waking life. If we have had an especially traumatic experience or even a difficult day, the dream material will be related to that experience, as the dream itself is a way of helping us to work through and face our anxieties in a more relaxed state of mind.

Based on that set of assumptions, participants in the workshop will, in the normal course of their dreaming experience, dream of any changes they are going through. By identifying a clear theme relating to this change ('Who am I as researcher?' 'What do I risk in my work?' 'Who am I after I retire?'), dreamers will be more aware of the issues involved in the change and therefore dream more vividly about this experience. Participating in SDD and having a theme related to the change they are experiencing often stimulates more dream material. Previous participants in SDD workshops report that their dream life increased as a result of the experience.

How to identify an appropriate theme is the next question. In my experience, it is occasionally helpful to ask participants at an orientation session to consider different themes, or at least to ask them to talk about the transitional experience they are going through. Sometimes the theme can be identified then. If not, usually the material shared in the introductory session can help the facilitator propose a suitable theme.

As mentioned, I always phrase the theme as a question, because a key issue can be embedded in the question without it being too confrontational. It is a question to consider, not a statement to agree with. For example, a theme such as 'Who am I after I retire?' reflects a deeply difficult life challenge for many people, but it suggests, at the same time, that I can be someone else. There is hope as well as worry embedded in the question.

Assembling a group

As will now be clear, SDD is a method recommended particularly for people going through major life transitions. How one recruits these participants and how one 'sells' potential recruits the benefits of this method are important practical questions.

Sharing dreams and drawings is not for everyone. This workshop is appropriate only for those who have the capacity, curiosity and willingness to partake in a creative and unknown process aimed at supporting them in their development. This is a workshop for those who voluntarily engage with it and who have an interest in the process. It should not be a required activity as part of any professional development, degree or outplacement programme. However, it could function very well as one option among others for advanced or expanded learning. It would also be appropriate for those who are already working together and going through a similar change, and who want to go more deeply into their own learning.

The marketing of such a workshop, whether by an email invitation, Facebook posting or a flyer on the wall, should include the following basic information:

Name of the method: Social Dream-Drawing
Name and title of facilitator:
Brief description of the method: participants in SDD share drawings of recent dreams and work as a group to link the meaning of these dreams to their current life changes.

Purpose of the workshop: to help participants develop strategies to cope well with a current life change.

Brief description of what current research says about dreaming: e.g. that dreams are vehicles for solving problems and for offering creative alternatives to the conscious mind in times of challenge and change.

Suggested dates and place:

Time frame:

Facilitator contact information:

The theme for this workshop is: e.g. 'How do I envision my future?'

Fee:

Deadline for contact:

Where possible, it's a good idea to hold an open orientation session for those interested. Here one can explain the method, outline the time constraints and ground rules and answer questions of concern. It might even be possible to work with a dream drawing that someone has brought along, to introduce people to the method.

One key issue is how many participants to include in a workshop. Since the work is so intense and usually 45 minutes to an hour is devoted to each dream drawing, there is a limit to how many people can participate, assuming everyone brings a dream drawing to each session. At the maximum, I have worked with groups of six people and, at the minimum, groups of three. I would say from experience that four or five is the ideal number. There needs to be enough participants to offer rich associations, but not so few that each dream drawer feels too much in the spotlight. As one London participant noted: 'It was a little bit more varied and rich as a result of having four people rather than three'.

That said, I have also conducted SDD workshops with a larger group of people. Sometimes people are interested in learning about the method, but are not themselves ready to bring their dream drawings. As previously mentioned, in an online training session for those interested in being certified in the method, I worked with a group of ten participants. Four of them worked with one dream drawing, and the others observed. When it came to the reflection session, we discovered that the observers had important insights into the theme. As a result of this learning, I now conduct SDD with larger groups. I divide them into the group working directly with the dream drawing and the group observing the process. This has the great advantage of expanding the number of participants and giving more richness to the learning.

At the end of this chapter, I will describe a recent online variation of SDD where participants were divided into three groups.

When it comes to forming the group, it is recommended that facilitators only accept those who are able to commit in advance to attending all the sessions. One of the key factors in the success of SDD is the working relationship that develops between the participants over time. And, obviously, the longer the group meets over the time, the more significant the learning and the deeper the connections between those taking part.

Once the group has been formed, I recommend sending each person a letter of confirmation with significant details of the upcoming workshop. Here is one example:

Dear Evelyn, Gary, John and Francis:

I am delighted that we will be working together on Tuesday, July 4th from 9:30 to 16:30 in a Social Dream-Drawing workshop. The theme for this workshop will be 'Who am I in this staff group?'

I invite each of you to bring a drawing of a dream. We will work for an hour on each dream drawing. During this hour, we will offer our free associations and amplifications to the drawing and then switch gears to reflect together on the theme.

Here are the six steps in the process:

Step 1: Dreamer tells the dream (3 to 5 minutes)
Step 2: Dreamer shows and explains the drawing (3 to 5 minutes)
Step 3: Participants ask clarifying questions of the dream drawer (3 to 5 minutes)
Step 4: All of us (including the dreamer and myself) offer free associations and amplifications (15 to 20 minutes)
Step 5: Dreamer responds to free associations; discussion follows (5 to 10 minutes)
Step 6: We reflect on the theme (15 to 20 minutes)

In case you consider it a challenge to remember and then to draw your dreams, here are a few recommendations.

Most of the richest dreams take place shortly before we wake up, so if you can anticipate this on those days when it is possible to 'sleep in', you will have plenty of dream material available.

When you realise you have had a dream, don't move! Believe it or not, dream material can quickly slip away when we change our body position. Thus, it is a good idea (if possible) to have a pad and drawing materials easily available from any position. Try to sit up and move slowly to get in position to draw.

Use any drawing materials and paper that you like. Colour or black and white is fine.

When it is possible, it is very interesting to begin your drawing before the inevitable phase of remembering the details. Social Dream-Drawing is based on the fact that dreams are in fact visual, and drawings can capture much of the primitive material that a verbal explanation cannot.

The extent to which there is a minimum of time, interruption, or movement between the dream experience and the drawing, the better.

Some of you may have long extended dreams. There are different ways of capturing these dreams. Some people use a different sheet of paper for each 'chapter' of their dream. Others just divide a single piece of paper into different segments. What also works very well is to draw one strong image from the entire dream. Usually that is a helpful prompt for the dreamer to remember the entire dream. Even a small dream fragment can suffice for a dream drawing.

Please don't worry about how good your drawing is or how realistic it is. The elements of the drawing are the catalysts for our free associations. For purposes of our work, the important thing is to bring a visual representation that can serve as a 'third object' for our exploration.

Although the workshop is a few weeks away, I suggest you begin right away to draw your dreams. This is a 'practice' that becomes more and more familiar when one undertakes it over a period of time.

Perhaps you will have many dreams and many dream drawings. You are free to bring whichever one you want to the workshop. This dream drawing does not have to appear to have any connection to the theme. Just bring the drawing that you most want to share and work with.

And, by the way, if you don't have a dream drawing by the time that we meet in the first session, don't worry. Sometimes it is better to work with fewer dreams in session one. However, your dream drawings will eventually be needed, so please keep trying!

After the workshop, if you are interested, I can send you an article I have published about the Social Dream-Drawing methodology. In general, I prefer that participants first have the experience before reading literature.

Please contact me if you have any further questions.

Lastly, looking forward so much to being with you in your dream worlds!

Warm regards, Rose

One of the most common reservations that people have to participate in SDD is that they say they don't dream. However, interestingly, even a letter like the one above can change that situation. Frederick in the London group noted: 'It was interesting that I haven't really dreamt until this week .... but this week I suddenly had dreamt because I knew I was coming here and it's almost like it is in the mind really .... it sort of freed me and for three nights I dreamt in a row'. And once people participate, they find they dream even more.

Confidentiality

The general rule of thumb, as all professionals and many readers of this book will know, is that when there is a group experience of any kind where people share deeply personal experiences, there needs to be a general agreement that whatever is shared in this space is not talked about to anyone outside of the group. In general, it is often only necessary for people to give their verbal promise that they will keep the material confidential. This verbal agreement can be given either in the introductory session or in the first workshop, before the work itself begins.

Keeping to this confidentiality rule is especially important when working with sub-groups that are part of a larger organisation. Information leaked from such a group can not only have direct consequences on colleagues, but may shatter the trust between group members and therefore undermine the work of the group as a whole.

The general exception to this rule, which was the case for me, is if you are using the material as part of your research for either a doctoral degree or future publication, in which case you should ask participants to sign a consent form. Because I was also recording the sessions, I used a special consent form that was attached to an extensive letter outlining the purpose of the group and explaining how it fitted in with my doctoral studies.

Another form of confidentiality is to forbid group members to discuss what has taken place within the group outside of the group space. This way, the work stays in the group where it belongs.

There are important reasons for prohibiting such discussions, which at first might not always be so apparent to group members. In workshops where participants may feel vulnerable and exposed, it is always tempting to try to find an ally, who will somehow protect us. Once such an alliance is created, the dynamic of this pairing will impact the work of the group. For example, one of them might only offer positive associations to a drawing or make positive comments about the other. Or both participants could agree not to participate at all. These and other possible consequences all hinder the free flow of associative thought.

The exception might be if a key topic has already been explored in the group (such as fears of bankruptcy), which is then discussed by the pair outside it. That can be an appropriate way of extending the learning to our real world. However, if the pair instead focuses on the inadequacies or the weakness of other group members who fear bankruptcy, then an alliance has already formed between them that will be enacted at the next session.

This does not mean that group members (who often already know one another) should not meet in between sessions. It is actually hoped that trusting and supporting relationships will develop from the group experience. But the nature of the conversation is what is important. Two friends in the London group, for example, met between sessions. Although at times, the topic of their individual transition experiences came up in the conversation (doing a doctorate and moving from Ireland to London), they were careful not to refer to what actually took place in the group. That is the desired norm here.

The physical space

There are many factors to consider when choosing an appropriate venue in which to hold the workshop. Before exploring issues regarding the physical setting, I want to discuss the overriding factors relating to this choice.

Much about the decision of location has to do with the nature of the workshop in relation to the needs of the group. For example, if the workshop is being offered to students doing a PhD, who perhaps travel quite a distance to attend seminars and lectures, it makes sense to hold the event in an empty classroom at the university. If, on the other hand, the workshop is to be offered as part of an outplacement programme, it makes sense to hold it somewhere that is physically separate from the workplace, in order to maintain privacy and symbolise a separation from the workplace.

In an SDD workshop, participants become vulnerable, as they are exploring their worries and challenges in relation to their current transition. Above all, they must feel they are in a safe place, what management professor John Newton has described as a 'sanctuary',[1] a place where one feels good being inside of it. Any setting that involves regular intrusions (people coming in and out, the pinging of emails, loud traffic, etc.) is to be avoided. Convenience and solace are prime factors.

I myself have facilitated this sort of workshop in many different settings, e.g. conference centres, university classrooms, living rooms, dining rooms, and office spaces. The decision needs to make sense to the participants and be linked to the defining transitional issue they are working on. Neither an overly formal and official setting, nor an overly informal setting is appropriate. A smaller, as opposed to a larger room, is to be preferred.

As to the physical setting itself, there are two primary configurations. One is a small table surrounded by chairs or a group of chairs placed in a small circle, with enough space in the middle for the drawings to be laid out. In the second instance, where there is no table, a rug is helpful, as it keeps the drawing itself clean and thus represents respect for it.

Figure 4.1 shows two settings in which I have conducted SDD workshops. Note the elements that offer structure (the arrangement of chairs, a centre point and adequate lighting) and those that offer a sense of comfort (window view, soft colours, paintings on the wall). Both of these settings capture the desired atmosphere for thoughtful work.

As explained in the next chapter, it is also a great advantage to have either a whiteboard or a flip chart available. On it, the schedule for the workshop and the six steps of the workshop can be written out. Having these parameters plainly available offers a sense of safety and security to participants and to the facilitator!

If one is holding a series of workshops over a period of time, the room itself takes on the function of offering a sense of security. As one London participant noted in her interview during the course of my research: 'There

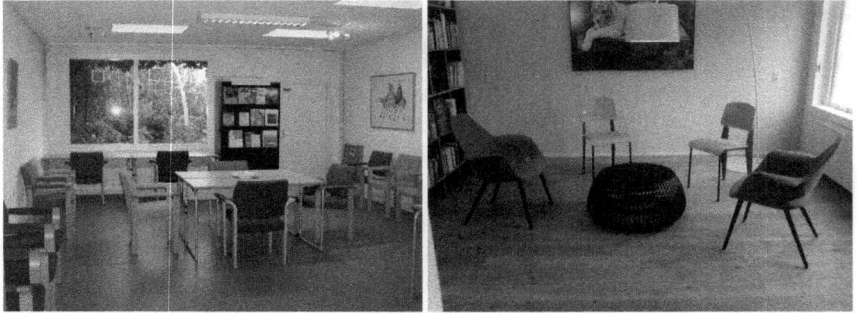

Figure 4.1 Settings for Social Dream-Drawing workshops

is something comforting about knowing that you're going to the same room'. It is preferable to find a space that may otherwise have many uses, but becomes identified by the participants as their workshop space. The same goes, by the way, for choosing the same time of day and perhaps day of the week. Anything that promotes familiarity between and during sessions is helpful to the process.

Single or multiple workshops?

It is important to note at this point that most of the impact of an SDD workshop takes place after the event is over. This can occur on the way home by car, or the next day at work, or even years later, as participants have told me in interviews. The experience takes time to be integrated and thought about. Thus it can be very helpful to organise a series of workshops over an extended period of time, perhaps over the course of a year and a half.

There are, of course, grounds for doing just one workshop. One critical factor has to do with travel and distance. For my doctoral research, I held only one workshop in Chile and one in South Africa, while I was able to manage multiple workshops in London, the Netherlands and Germany.

For a group that is stuck on a particular issue relating to the change they are experiencing, a SDD workshop might be suggested simply in order to investigate it at a deeper level. Perhaps one workshop will be enough. Or it could lead to requests for more.

If multiple workshops are to be held, it is important that the sessions are spaced close enough in time, so that a sense of connection can develop between participants. But they should also be far enough apart that participants have enough time to integrate the experience. It is also recommended that you do not schedule all the sessions in advance, but arrange them workshop by workshop, to accommodate the complications of people's busy lives.

One need, which is often not recognised at first, is for an ongoing support system during a major time of change. Multiple SDD workshops provide this. London research participant Deidre put it this way: 'Probably one of the objective attractions to doing this as well, is that it allowed me to maintain contact with people who think in this way, or are open to viewing the world with this perspective'.

Dream drawings brought to a session versus those drawn during the session

In 2013, I co-hosted an SDD workshop with my colleague Simon Turner. In our discussions, we realised that those dream drawings that were drawn after the theme was announced led to the most vibrant and intense work. As Bollas points out, although a dream may contain 'an infinite web of meanings',[2] there is a context and an inherent task in SDD, i.e. to manage a transition.

Dream drawings of recurring dreams or an important dream from the past are never easy to work with in a workshop setting, because these are not specifically connected to or stimulated by the identified theme. While the dream may have a special meaning for the dreamer, its underlying material makes it more of a personal dream than a social dream. That is not to say it is a bad dream or a bad drawing, only that it is not the best material for the workshop.

Sometimes participants ask if they can draw the dream after they have arrived. We have found this to be problematic. The problem here is that once one enters the workshop space and interacts with others, whatever is drawn is one way or another influenced by the group dynamic. It is a drawing that is not done in the quiet, reflective space of immediately recalling a dream experience. It is often quite superficial and only depicts major events, not the usual subtleties of a dream drawing.

In contrast to this perspective, colleagues of mine (see Chapter 10) have been using SDD as an organisational diagnostic tool. This is when someone mentions that they have had a dream, and the supervisor asks them to draw the dream then and there. In this case, as my colleague put it, 'the drawing is influenced by this felt relatedness to the group', and therefore makes available more valuable unconscious group data.

During an online SDD workshop, sponsored by an international organisation, one participant expressed her interest in drawing the dreams of others. She wondered aloud what might be learned from such a method. Intrigued by this idea, my colleague Anton Zemlyanoy and I organised and ran an online workshop pilot programme in the fall of 2021. We invited recent graduates of the Psychoanalytic Executive Coaching Master's Program at the National Research University: Higher School of Economics in Moscow to attend. Our theme was 'Dreaming the future of me as a Professional Consultant and Coach'.

Although all participants were asked to bring (or have available to show) dream drawings, we only worked with one dream and its drawing during

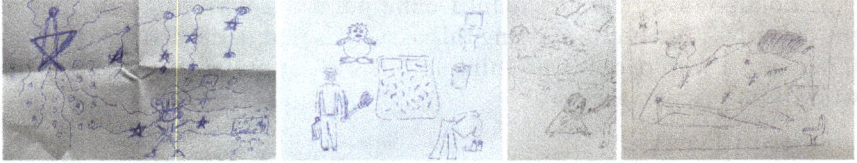

Figure 4.2 Drawing other people's dreams

each session. Before seeing the drawing of the dreamer, members of the group were asked to draw this dream as it was being told. Figure 4.2 shows three drawings of Martha's dream by other participants, followed by Martha's own drawing of her dream, which she shared with us afterwards.

We discovered that when participants draw the dreams of others, the variety of visual images and free associations are greatly expanded. These pre-verbal responses to the told dream made space for the unconscious associative material of participants to be seen and worked with. As such, the original dream material becomes more and more reflective of and relevant to the whole group's transitional experience.

We also learned that by dividing up the group into three separate sub-groups, there was very rich reflection and learning.[3] Very important themes were identified and discussed in depth. These included how to integrate their new learning into their previous work and the various barriers to their starting an independent consulting practice.

Having summarised the essential elements to keep in mind when planning to offer an SDD workshop, I would like us to turn next to the experience of the workshop itself. Now the participants have been selected, the room has been identified, a flip chart or a whiteboard stand ready, and people have dream drawings in their hands ...

Notes

1 Newton, J. (1999) Clinging to the MBA syndicate: shallowness and 'Second Skin' learning in management education. *Socio-Analysis.* 1(2), p. 156.
2 Bollas, C. (2011) *The Christopher Bollas Reader.* London: Routledge, p. 251.
3 I recommend this article for further elucidation of this concept: Morgan-Jones, R.J. (2022 forthcoming) The Trilogy Matrix Event: a setting for integrating the study of large social system dynamics from different dimensions. In: Hopper, E. & Weinberg, H., eds., *The Social Unconscious in Persons, Groups and Societies: Clinical Implications – Volume 4.* London: Routledge.

Chapter 5

Conducting a Social Dream-Drawing workshop

In the previous chapter, we looked in depth at the factors that go into organising and undertaking a Social Dream-Drawing (SDD) workshop. However, before we get into the details of the event itself, I want to share with you some insights into how, despite all of the preparation, things can still go wrong.

Even with all the preparation in the world, the first meeting of a group always brings with it a sense of uncertainty and anxiety. Not just for the participants but for the facilitator as well. This happened to me, when I held my first research group in London. The stakes couldn't have been higher, because this was the first native English-speaking group that I had worked with. I had to audio record the session and came equipped with the latest recording device. Frederick was ready to share his dream drawing with us. And then I panicked.

Although I had practised endlessly with this new gizmo at home, I couldn't figure out how to get it going. And so the whole emotional charge of starting this new experience had to be put on pause, while Frederick helped me figure out which buttons to push and how to start recording.

Sadly, we were both wrong. During this first most wonderful session, which I enjoyed so much and in which the group participated so actively, I did not press record correctly, and we have no recording of it. To this day, I deeply regret this mistake, which I can only offer to you, dear reader, as an example of all the unconscious anxieties that relate to entering the unconscious realm of dream drawings.

Sharing the schedule

Before the participants enter the room where the workshop is to take place, the furniture should be set out as described previously, i.e. chairs set in a circle around either a small table or around sufficient floor space to display the dream drawings. When possible at this stage, the schedule should be clearly written by the facilitator on a whiteboard or a flip chart. This should remain in view during the course of the session so that participants can easily refer to it.

DOI: 10.4324/9780429275647-6

The mere act of writing out the schedule (as opposed to the facilitator having it only in his or her head) communicates to the participants that there will be an orderly progression to the day. Although the dream material itself requires a kind of timeless attention, the schedule holds the day together. A schedule placed in full view of everyone offers a sense of structure to the participants, many of whom will not have participated in a workshop like this before.

Deirdre, a participant in my London research workshop, noted how useful it was to have the schedule to hand in this way:

> I think there's a sense that it's very clear how long I'm going to be here, how long I'm going to be expected to speak about my piece of work, how long I'm going to be expected to listen to others' feedback and so on. And I think that creates safety, but I also think it maintains interest because I guess we don't know how long a conversation might go on for. Will I get bored and think 'oh God this could go on for three hours about one topic,' rather than saying we have three hours and this is how we're going to use it? I think for me [a schedule] helps maintain interest in the process.

Having a written schedule also communicates to participants that they will have only a certain amount of time and space for their drawing. Thus, participants know they will have to organise their presentations to fit this time frame. Fran, another participant in the London research group, put it this way: 'If you know as participant how much time there is going to be on your drawing, then people have an innate sense to get … what they need out from it'.

The workshop begins with a review of the schedule. At this point, group members decide whose dream drawing will be worked on at which time, so there are no surprises as the day proceeds. Generally, those who are the most unsure of the experience will ask to go later and, if possible, this should be accommodated.

If it turns out that there is not enough time for each dream drawing to be worked on for an hour, then adjustments can now be made to ensure that each participant has an equal amount of time for his or her drawing. The main point is not to short-change anyone in terms of time spent on the dream drawings they have brought to the session.

It may be the case that some participants show up without a drawing. Under these circumstances, the schedule can be adjusted in any number of ways. One can allow more time for working with the individual dream drawings that have been brought to the session. One can extend a coffee or a lunch break or even decide to end the workshop early. Another option is to engage in a general discussion of how the workshop has impacted everyone and what feedback they may want to give to the facilitator. With SDD, there is never the problem of having too much time!

If offering multiple workshops, a good rule of thumb is to begin the next session with the question of whether there is any material left over from the previous workshop that participants want to bring up and discuss. This could include further thoughts on a topic that was discussed last time (such as how one's writing block on one's dissertation seems to have gone away or – as was my personal experience – how work on a dream drawing relating to a client helped me develop more empathy for her). Sometimes participants want to bring up something that happened in the group during the last session, such as a feeling of having been criticised for making simple drawings. It's very important that these kinds of issues are aired, otherwise the fear of being criticised, for example, will influence this person's future work in the group, and thus inhibit free association and free drawing. This review task should be given a slot of about ten minutes at most on the written schedule.

The written schedule does not have to be the most professional presentation, but it has to be clear. It's a good idea to have the name of each participant written in the order that they will share his or her dream drawing.

Another point about creating a schedule is to build in a pause between working on each individual dream drawing. Fifteen minutes often does the trick. This allows for a quick bathroom break, but also – especially for the dream drawer whose picture was the last subject of the session – a chance to reflect. This work requires quite a bit of concentration and effort, and participants will need to take regular breaks from these demands.

In addition to writing out the day's structure in advance, I always write down the six steps of the workshop, so that participants can easily orient themselves when we are working on a drawing. This again demonstrates that SDD is a well thought-out process. The overall theme of the workshop is also written and displayed, as a clear reminder of the focus of the work.

In facilitating an SDD workshop, it is always essential to follow a consistent structure. This creates comfort, predictability and safety. It is not necessary for the participants to understand why the structure is what it is. What is important is that it doesn't vary. As Frederick, the participant in that first London research group, noted:

> I liked the structure of it and the moving around. I didn't often understand what we were doing, but it felt well thought through ... I didn't get the sense that we were jumping backwards and to other things. It did feel that the boundary was set physically, so you could do the next bit. It was very good and overall felt very well thought through.

The first session

When offering multiple workshops, sometimes it is worth holding an orientation session before the work begins in earnest on the drawings. This gives the participants a chance to get to know one another, which is a great advantage for those meeting for the first time. In such a first session, you could, for instance, lead a small activity related to drawing that allows the participants to become comfortable with one another. For example, for a group in Germany, I asked people to draw a picture related to our theme of 'What do I risk in my work?' Later, they shared these pictures with one another. Figure 5.1 shows one example.

In this drawing, Christine drew her dilemma as a university professor. She explained that she had felt boxed in by all the requirements of her university work (the three brown boxes), while she saw herself as creative and colourful and was looking for a way out of the system to express this side of her personality. As previously described in Chapter 1, this dilemma of transitioning out of the university (she was shortly eligible for retirement) became the primary theme of her work in the SDD sessions. At the end of them, she realised that the university had actually promoted her creativity in ways she hadn't appreciated (see the extensive discussion of the bakehouse dream shown in Figure 1.1).

In addition to a getting-to-know-you exercise, an orientation session gives participants the opportunity to ask the facilitator questions about the method. The facilitator can give clear instructions on how to do dream drawing at home as well. And if it is not possible to hold an orientation session, then a detailed letter is very helpful (see the example in Chapter 4).

In the first session in which dream drawings are worked on, the schedule may require a certain amount of flexibility. In the London group, a colleague helped support my role as facilitator. She observed that it might be better if fewer dreams were worked on in the first session, so that people

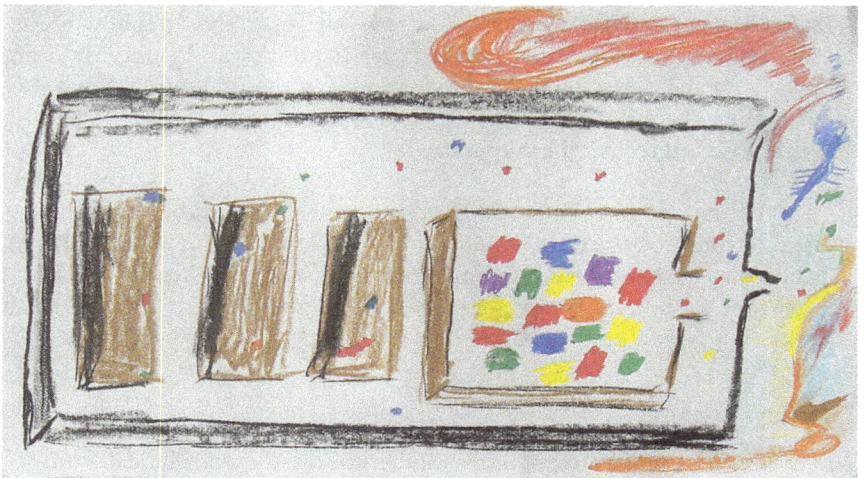

Figure 5.1 Orientation meeting drawing

could familiarise themselves with the process and the time pressure was not so great. One participant in this group suggested that: 'In a future session you might want to allow a little bit of extra time in the first session to allow the explanation and the forming to happen. And then for subsequent sessions you could move that time'.

The dream drawings are then worked on one at a time. This means that when people arrive at the session with their drawings, they are not tempted to share them with others at this point, as they know that the picture will be worked on later during the session itself. With this temptation in mind, it is a good idea to have a handy place for participants to place their drawings when they are not in use.

The six steps in Social Dream-Drawing

What follows now are specific directions for working with each individual dream drawing. It is important here to emphasise that for many participants, this process will be a completely unfamiliar experience. Most people don't really know how to free associate, for example. Many people at first confuse clarifying questions with offering interpretations of the drawings (see Step 3, below). That is normal. What is important is that the facilitator remains consistent, giving the same directions and examples to everybody. Over time, participants will learn the various skills, just as they will learn the skill of doing a dream drawing itself. So for the first session, the facilitator may need to be especially active and attentive until participants understand the task required by each step.

When meeting in person, I try to sit next to the person who is presenting his dream drawing, to offer a sense of support and connection when necessary.

Step 1: Dream drawer describes the dream (3 to 5 minutes)

As previously mentioned, we begin by having the dreamer first describe the dream, e.g. 'Okay, John, can you please tell us about your dream?' The reason for this is to help the dreamer return as much as possible to the original dream experience by describing it to others, and also to encourage the other participants to form images in their own heads in anticipation of seeing the drawing. This is an easy entry into the dream material.

Step 2: Dream drawer shows and explains the drawing (3 to 5 minutes)

The facilitator asks the dreamer to show us the drawing: 'Can you please now show us your drawing of this dream?' He then places the drawing on the table or the floor, facing himself. Some participants may view the drawing 'upside down', but that actually frees up people to offer associations from other visual perspectives. I ask the dreamer to explain the drawing: 'Okay, can you please tell us about your drawing?' As drawings range from the most basic to the most complicated, this can take some time. The dream drawer is free to speak without interruption until he is finished.

Step 3: Participants ask clarifying questions of the dream drawer (3 to 5 minutes)

At this point, other participants have an opportunity to clarify for themselves those parts of the drawings that they didn't quite understand. They may ask the dream drawer to say something about a certain image that was not mentioned, for example, or ask the dream drawer to repeat something that wasn't understood earlier. These questions address matters of clarification that, unless articulated, might somehow impede the participants' ability to begin work in earnest on the drawing.

This is a tricky step, because there is a very fine line between a question whose answer clarifies something and a question in which a hypothesis or an interpretation is imbedded. For example, when someone asks the dream drawer, 'Why is there so much free space in your drawing?' there is a judgement being made. The questioner is somehow suggesting that this drawing is not finished, for example. This asks the dream drawer to attempt to justify his work, and that is not the point of this phase.

When such a question arises, it is important for the facilitator to remind participants of this issue, for example: 'At the moment, we are only seeking the clarification of information, not explanations of decisions'. For some participants, this is a particularly difficult learning to integrate, and facilitators must stay consistent on this point. It is important to keep these questions focused and at a minimum in order for the other participants to feel they can begin to work.

Step 4: All of us (including the dreamer and facilitator) offer free associations and amplifications to the dream drawing (15 to 20 minutes)

This step is pretty much the bread and butter of the method: 'Okay, everyone. Now that we have had a chance to hear John describe his dream and explain his dream drawing, I want to ask you all for your free associations to this material. This means saying whatever springs to mind, no matter how crazy or inappropriate it may at first sound'.

As has been mentioned, not everyone can free associate to begin with. Interpretations ('It looks to me as if the dreamer does not like cows') or direct questions to the dream drawer ('Why did you draw that green?') are common missteps that put the focus on the person drawing and interrupt the free flow of ideas and associations. The drawing is the focus, not the dream drawer. Free associations and amplifications are the expressions of the creative and uncensored mind, and they take practice.

Often one person's associations stimulate another's associations. That is quite normal. Sometimes the associations are hilarious. Sometimes a bit sexy. As thoughts from the unconscious, they are not supposed to follow some sort of logic (see Chapter 3). They are offered to free up the dreamer and group members, allowing them to discover other meanings from the dream material.

The facilitator is also free to associate, but must keep in mind that, as with all groups, the person in the role of leader is the top person in the hierarchy, and that person's free associations can influence the others (the role of the facilitator is discussed in depth in Chapter 8). When the leader is too active or offers the first associations, there is a danger that group members, in their desire to perform well, will imitate him or her. When that happens, their own original associations will be lost.

The dreamer is also encouraged to free associate. Over time I have learnt that this can be a great opportunity for the dreamer to return once more to the dream experience, where new dream material comes forth, especially in response to the associations of others in the group. I have described a good example of this in Chapter 2, regarding the red cross on the bed.

As noted above, I recommend allowing 15–20 minutes for this phase; however, this is not always necessary. For many groups, spending so much time on each dream drawing may seem excessive. One really has to judge the tolerance of a group for the amount of time allocated.

When it appears that a group really has no more to offer during the time allocated for free-association, it is perfectly fine to end this phase and extend the reflective phase that follows. It could well be that such a drawing will serve as rich material for the reflection session and offer food for thought in different ways. As one London participant noted, when reflecting on her skimpy drawings:

> I would have [to] be quite honest, Rose, and say that when it came to drawing the drawing the day or two beforehand, or whenever I did it, I did it in probably five minutes … And that creates a question for me as to how slapdash maybe I am in my work, how much importance am I attaching, and [how] well do I prepare for presenting something …. What does that mean for my work in a wider context … am I a bit casual in [that] I'll get you something, but it [is] maybe not the richest thing that I will get you?

Then the opposite situation could occur. There are times when work on a single dream drawing cannot just end at the prescribed ending time according to the schedule. That is normal too. This means that the facilitator must allow for a bit of flexibility in conducting the workshop, but not so much flexibility that the core schedule is completely lost. There is a fine line between a flexible schedule and an unpredictable one. For those participants whose SDD are to be shared later on in the day, this is a particularly important issue.

As one London participant put it:

> It's important to have an agreed time boundary, with a couple minutes of flexibility in it. And I think that was handled quite well, we pretty much stuck to it, certainly my sense was that even if we were likely to exceed the limit time I knew. So let's just say there was a person with half an hour for their dream and at the end of the half an hour it was apparent that they wanted to go on for a bit longer. I didn't have a sense that we were going to run twenty minutes over into somebody else's half-hour. I had a sense they might go over for a minute or two, but just to let the conversation come to a natural conclusion.

Step 5: Dreamer responds to free associations; discussion follows (5–10 minutes)

Following the bread-and-butter segment of free associations by everyone, the dream drawer is given a chance to comment on the experience. It is no small thing to bring a drawing of a dream to a group and to make it available to everyone's spontaneous thoughts. A dream is a very private experience and not easily shared with others, much less in such an active and organised situation.

Very often, dream drawers are amazed at the associations offered by the other participants. Some comment on how much more of the dream came alive for them, in the sense that they brought to mind more dream material or that the associations really seemed to make sense of what the dream meant to them (see discussion and Figure 10.4 in Chapter 10 for my own example of this phenomenon).

Sometimes, however, the group work is not so easy for participants. One of the German group participants had missed the previous session, due to the imminent death of her husband. He died a few weeks later. She returned to the group for the next session, hoping to continue to work on her transitional issue, which had to do with a decision about retirement. She didn't want the group to focus on her mourning and grief over the loss of her husband. Instead, she wanted to focus on her retirement plans, so she was pleased that she 'had what I would call a normal interesting dream, with something happening, some scenery and so on' before the session. Figure 5.2 shows her drawing of that dream.

Unfortunately for her, however, there were many associations to death and danger. One participant said the dark brown structure looked like a

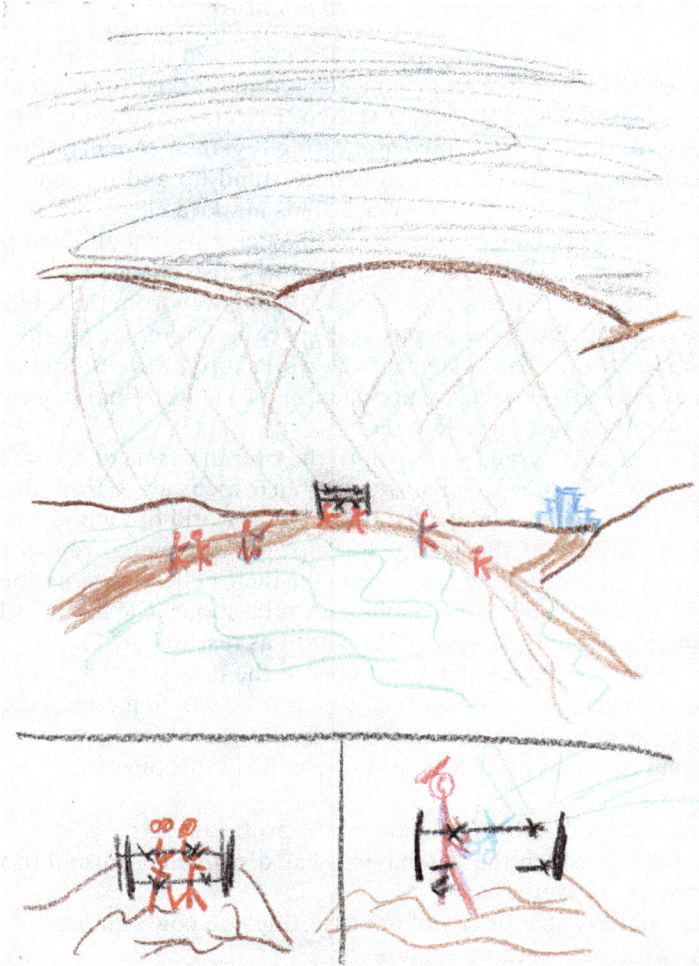

Figure 5.2 The gate

grave or a coffin. The dream drawer remembers quite vividly how difficult that was to hear. And unfortunately, there was no space in the schedule to give her a chance to talk about her emotional situation. When I thought about it after speaking with her, I think I erred in not making that space somehow possible.

To summarise then, this is an extremely important step, because it gives the dreamer the voice to respond and to express the strong feelings that are experienced when others are so intensively involved with his drawing. Sometimes it is revelation, sometimes it is anger … but mostly it is amazement!

Step 6: We reflect on the theme (15–20 minutes)

Up until this last step, the group has been immersed in the dream world in one way or another. But at this point, the group is asked to transition from this regressive state and to enter a state of reflection and thinking. This is not so easy to do. Therefore, when meeting together, to mark this change in consciousness, I ask group members to stand up and move to another seat, as described earlier, in Chapter 3. This marks a clear shift to another task and another state of mind, and puts participants in a different physical relationship to one another. As the facilitator, I also change my seat. When working online, we all take a two-minute break away from the screen.

This change in task and in physical space is reinforced in the written schedule setting out the six steps of the workshop. I always draw a strong line (usually in red) between the previous Step 5 and this final step to denote the change of task and consciousness.

Here, the group is asked to return to the overall theme of the workshop. They are asked, in other words, to move their focus away from the dream in which they have been immersed to the wider world of their current transition. The purpose of this step is to help group membes return to their 'real' worlds and to update themselves on their collective situation. They are asked to think about the theme and talk about it (e.g. 'So, what are your thoughts about our theme, "Who am I as researcher?"'). They are not asked to make a direct connection between the just-shared dream and the workshop's theme, only to talk about the theme itself. Sometimes the dream material enters the discussion and sometimes not.

Examples of topics that have been discussed in this phase are:

* The anxiety of taking up a new role as professor
* The ways in which the coronavirus has disrupted a normal process of transition into retirement
* An awareness of a history of not asserting one's own authority in situations with male authority figures
* The need to truly mourn the loss of a professional working partnership
* Those forces preventing a director from planning retirement from her current position
* The emotional longing for the physical environment one has left in relocating

Some participants have found this transitional stage quite difficult. One London participant felt strongly that the theme I used for her group ('What do I risk in my work?') was not really relevant to her, and thus this phase of the workshop was never going to be easy. She would have much preferred not to have had a theme at all or for the theme to have been developed with the group, and not imposed upon it by me. I found this to be very important feedback.

I continue to recommend using a theme, mostly because it helps the dreamers have a context for the dream material that they bring to the workshop. It helps narrow the focus and ensures the material specifically addresses a key transitional state.

Ending each workshop session

After all the dream drawings have been worked on, it is helpful to reflect together on the day's experiences. Although, by this point, the participants and facilitator are usually quite tired, it is important to give everyone the chance to raise any pressing issues they have and also to provide the facilitator with valuable feedback. To that end, the facilitator might say: 'For our last ten minutes today, I suggest we take some time to reflect on our overall experience of today's workshop. Are there any lingering concerns, comments or questions?'

It was during one of these reflective sessions with my London group, for example, that I received very positive comments on having the schedule and the flow of the workshop displayed on the wall. Up to then, I had not been so consistent in this practice, so this was very helpful.

This is also a good time to set the date for the next session. This final activity functions very well as an opportunity for everyone to transition back into daily life. People can say their goodbyes, assemble their personal belongings, and make their way out. From there, they have the time to reflect on what they have learnt and begin to anticipate the next time they will meet and work together.

Chapter 6

The final review session

The primary purpose of Social Dream-Drawing (SDD) is to impact people's lives in a meaningful and valuable way. As with any workshop experience, there is always the challenge of helping participants apply what they have learnt in a practical way to their daily professional and personal lives. I, therefore, recommend that after the last session in which a group actively works on new dream drawings, at least one, and perhaps two (see Chapter 7), review sessions be held. These two sessions provide participants with the opportunity to reflect on the entire experience and to conceptualise their learnings over this period of time. In a sense, each SDD session is a 'snapshot' of where participants are at that particular time. But bringing meaning to the whole experience can only take place once everything, in retrospect, is brought together.

There are a number of possible ways to glean meaning and overall insights from experience. In this chapter, I will be focusing on activities that help participants recognise the personal and individual meaning that the experience has had for them. (In Chapter 7, the focus will be on group learnings.) Here are three methods that can be combined in different ways to facilitate this integration and learning:

• Revisit the whole workshop by means of a group viewing of all the dream drawings
• Review of all the SDD sessions by means of printed transcripts
• Create individual timelines relating to the time span of the workshop

Revisit the whole workshop through a group viewing of all the dream drawings

The easiest and most direct way to help participants integrate their workshop experiences is by displaying the original dream drawings (or, when not available, photographs of these drawings) on the wall or on screen. They should be placed in chronological order. This means in the order they were worked on both in the session itself and in the order of the workshops over time. Displaying them will help participants immediately

DOI: 10.4324/9780429275647-7

recall their experiences (remember: drawings stay in the mind much longer than words).

The group can be asked first to view all of these drawings at a distance and to reflect on them and write down their impressions individually. Then the group can walk from drawing to drawing and discuss their reactions and memories. For such an exercise, one can simply remind participants of the dates and who did what drawing, if necessary. I have found that it doesn't take much. Participants enjoy revisiting these drawings and reminding themselves of the weather on that day or of some big event that had just occurred or was about to take place. This stage of the process doesn't need to be very strictly designed and can take about an hour.

For example, following an online SDD workshop, we viewed all four dream drawings at once on the screen. In Chapter 9 of this book, which describes this online workshop in detail, I discuss what this discussion entailed and what learnings came out of it.

Following such an examination of the images, participants can be asked to do some personal writing – a sort of individual free association. What did this exercise mean for them? What did they notice? What did it make them think about?

Following this individual work, the group can then reconvene and share these reactions and perceptions. Once a period of processing has taken place, the group can be asked to return, one last time, to the overall theme of the workshop. It might even be useful to ask them to do some individual thinking again about the theme before discussing it with the group as a whole. This last discussion could lead towards people identifying exactly what they have learnt for themselves that relates to the theme.

One notable example of such an insight comes from a Dutch group. At the time, I didn't set a theme for the workshops, so participants were not bringing drawings related to any particular set subject. In the case of one participant, he didn't realise what his theme was until the final review. Then he was able to identify a key professional anxiety he was experiencing as he neared the age of 60. He wanted to undertake a new way of consulting to organisations, but felt guilty about abandoning all that he had learnt as a young professional. The series of SDD workshops helped him to acknowledge what he had learnt and to move ahead without feelings of guilt.

Figure 6.1 shows the key dream drawing that represents this conflict.

Another variation on this design is to ask participants to put Post-it notes on the dream drawings that had the most meaning for them over the course of the workshops. They can identify as many as they like, and a discussion can ensue on why these particular drawings had so much meaning for them. This can then be directly related to the theme of the work.

All of these activities, then, are in relation to the drawings and the time span of the workshop. They give a chance for individual reflection as well as group discussion. They involve extensive individual reaction as well as

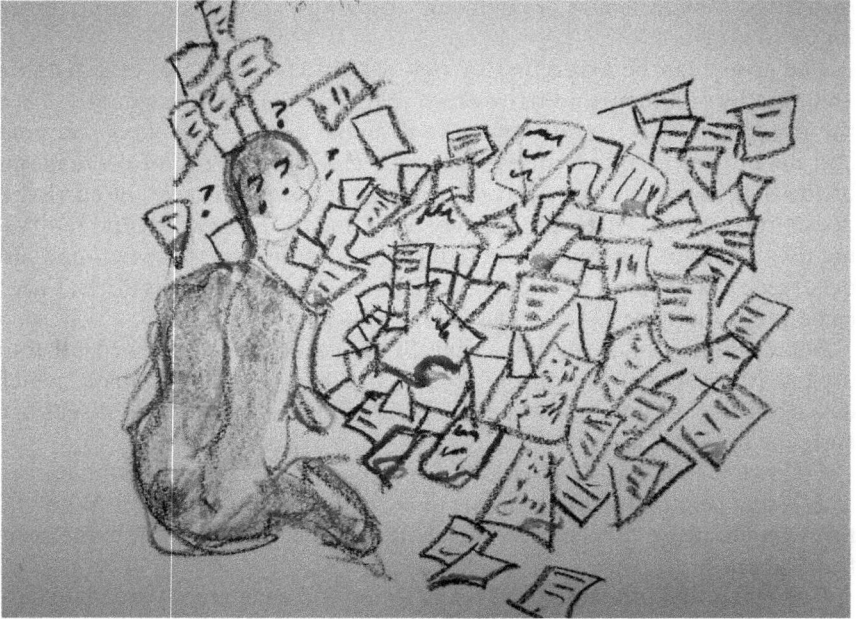

Figure 6.1 Letting go

group learning. It is almost always the case that, while participants may be working with the same theme, individual learnings vary from person to person. And this is the time to bring these learnings to mind.

Such a session can also provide space for thank yous and for a general discussion of the whole experience. Feedback to the facilitator can also be included.

Review of all SDD sessions by means of printed transcripts

For some groups that I have run over an extended period of time, I have distributed transcripts of each session to the participants between each session. As these face-to-face sessions can take place months apart, this is a way of keeping the work present in people's minds. (For an online workshop, where the sessions are not so far apart, this reminder may not be necessary. See Chapter 9.) While not all participants will read these transcripts between the sessions, the documents provide a very good way of helping people reflect on the workshop experience at the final review session.

There are different ways of producing transcripts. For the purposes of my doctoral work, which required reliable data for analysis, I taped each session myself and had them transcribed by a professional. Another way of making transcripts is to ask one person in each group to take notes for the session. So, for example, if there are four people in the group, each time a dream drawing is worked on, another member will take the notes. Then these roles rotate until everyone has had a chance to show a drawing and everyone has taken notes.

A third option is to have an outside recorder take notes. This was especially necessary when I ran SDD workshops in Chile when the dreamers spoke no English and I spoke no Spanish. The note-taker spoke both languages and recorded in both languages. Then she created an English version and a Spanish version. It was a great effort. The transcriber was allowed to participate in the associations and reflections.

Here, as an example, is the first page of a transcription of a session with the German group, translated into English:

Social Dream-Drawing
4th Session July 4, 2010
Solingen, Germany

Dreamers: Christine, Heike, Anna, Emre
Facilitator: Rose Mersky
Process Consultant: Heinz

Process

1 Dream Drawing
2 Questions
3 Associations and Amplifications
4 Response
5 Theme

Picture #1 (Figure 6.2): Christine
Note-taker: Anna

Christina's description of the dream: "'What is this all about?" I asked myself while writing it down. This dream took place in March 2010 in Lübeck. My dream about the bricks was earlier. There was a very spacious landscape, a golden, opulent landscape in summertime, all green and gold, with few people in sight. Then somebody says: "They are coming to attack us! They come from the background, from far off." At the same time: "How lovely!" "We've got to flee, in and up the tower!"... But it could only be a trick'.

For the last session of the German group, which met over a period of one and a half years in my home, I made copies of the transcripts for the participants. I took extensive notes on the day that we met to reflect on them, as follows:

I had printed out hard copies of our 4 previous sessions (Organising Meeting Sept. 26, 2009, First Dreaming and Drawing February 14, 2010, Second Dreaming and Drawing May 13, 2010 and Third Dreaming and Drawing July 4, 2010), which were on the table. Plus I brought my own

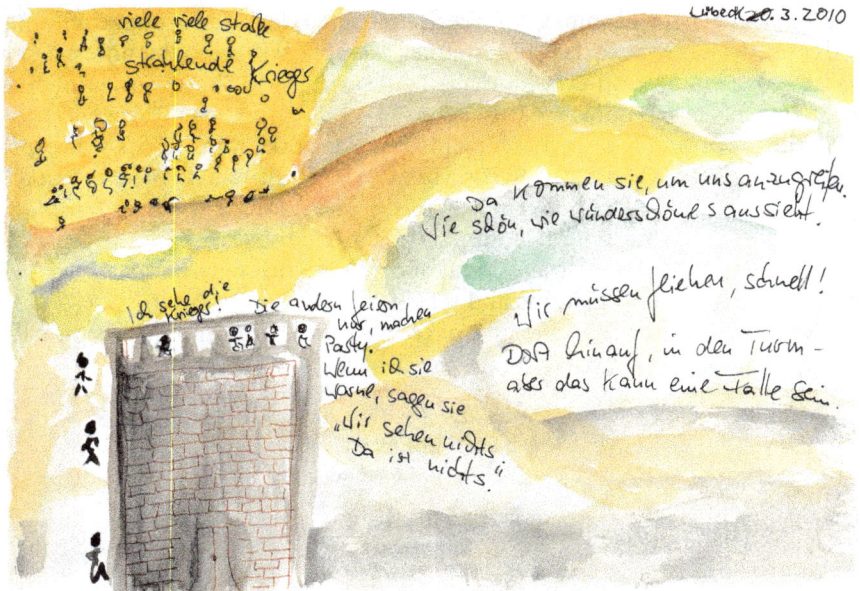

Figure 6.2 The tower

2009, 2010 and 2011 calendars …. We began to look through the transcripts of the 4 previous sessions and reviewed each participant's drawings over the time of our work together. These transcripts became a kind of 'living gold' as they were checked and reviewed again and again.

Together, using the transcripts I had made available, the four participants reviewed each person's dreams in the order they were dreamt and shared in the group. What surprised me was that the transcripts demonstrated to the participants how well-organised I actually was in conducting this workshop:

> Then Anna laid out the transcripts on the table, so that they could see how much time had elapsed between the sessions. They realised then that I had always had a particular plan for our work together and that the weather and illnesses had somehow interceded. I had the impression that they appreciated that I had the transcripts available for them to remember their history and that I really had had a plan in my mind. Somehow I think this made them realise that this experience, in which they had been immersed, had been well contained and planned by me.

This activity could easily be followed by some of the steps mentioned above, such as personal responses in a journal which are then shared with the group. Combining a review of the transcripts with the first activity, i.e. the joint viewing, may be too much, so one or the other activity is recommended. While both activities allow for a free review of events, I would say that the transcripts remind the participants of more of the details and perhaps offer more insight into the theme.

Create individual timelines relating to the time span of the workshop

In order to deepen the connection between the experiences in the individual workshop sessions and the important events in the participants' lives and in the world during this same time, I ask participants to create a personal timeline. To facilitate this, participants are asked to enter data relating to certain categories.

A German group agreed to take their personal information and enter it into a collective timeline (see Chapter 7). Thus, before they could start their personal timelines, they had to decide what the time boundaries were for the experience. As it turned out, there were not only significant differences between the personal timelines themselves. Participants also had different views about them. As a result, this proved to be a very difficult request, but one that in itself brought insight. As I wrote at the time:

> One of the first questions was, what should the end point of our timeline be or how far into the future should it go. They had a major and long discussion about the future, i.e. in thinking about this experience, how does it relate to some future event. It was obvious that it would be different for each one of them. In other words, each of them was customising the experience according to his/her own development. For Heike, for example, it was definitely about helping her make the transition to leaving her school role, which she will do in one and a half years' time. For Anna, it started as a process of deciding whether to take retirement in five years or in ten years, but it all changed when her husband died in the middle of our work .... For Emre, he absolutely couldn't concretise the idea of time and the future. He couldn't see that this particular experience might have helped in a particular way to work through something, even though it was during this one and a half years [September 26, 2009 to March 20, 2011] that he finished the first draft of his doctoral thesis.

Creating their personal timelines absorbed the group.

Why did I choose this activity? Over the course of a long series of SDD workshops, it is only normal that major events will have taken place both in the personal lives of the participants and on the world stage as well. While these important events sometimes appear in the dream material, quite often, they stand separate from the focus of the workshop and thus are not fully integrated into the work.

One major example of this was the concern of one London member that he had cancer (he didn't) and the ongoing illness of the son of another group member. Neither of them had spoken of these major life concerns in our group meetings. Our focus was elsewhere. It was only possible and appropriate to share these experiences in the course of compiling the timeline, where they were encouraged to connect our work with events in their individual lives.

I began to wonder, for example, how one participant's health concerns would affect his ability to take risks in his work environment. Or whether the global financial crisis would affect PhD students concerned about financing such a major endeavour as their studies. Would they risk pursuing a particularly limited research goal, knowing that funding for that particular area might not be available in the future? Or, for the principal of an elementary school forced to move location due to a collapse in the neighbouring infrastructure, how much could she risk pushing her teachers to develop new ways of teaching in the classroom? Where did the limits of possibility lie?

Here my goal was to help them expand their explorations of risk in their work in relation to their actual work situations and challenges.

This activity had the effect of helping each participant think about his or her individual future. Thus it served as an excellent transitional experience out of the workshop. It was amazing how seriously participants took this task and how meaningful it was. As I wrote at the time: 'It's great to see their concentration and the way they are thinking all of this through. Integrating this experience,

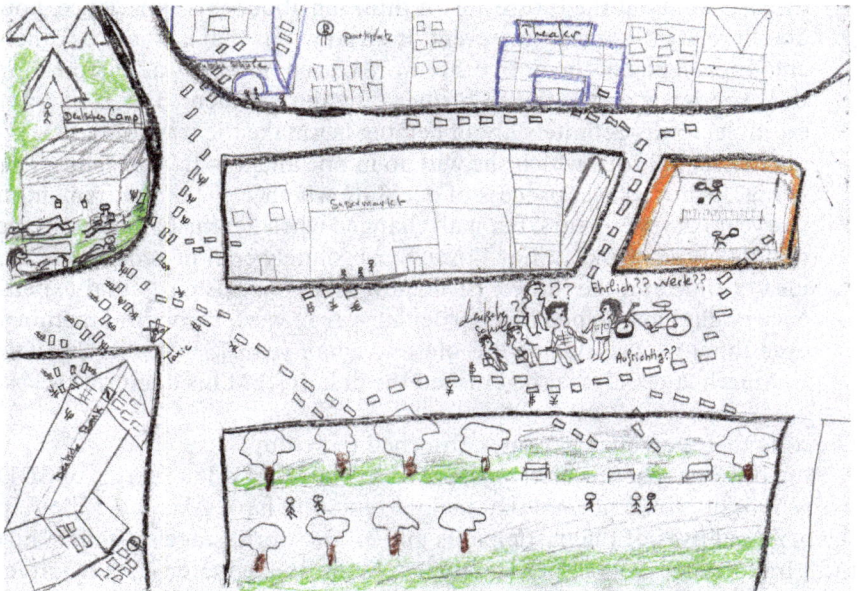

Figure 6.3 Lost in a German city

thinking about the last year and a half'. At this point, they could articulate clear concepts about what direction they were going and when. At least, this was true of the three participants in the German group who were facing decisions about retirement.

The fourth participant was much younger and just starting his doctoral studies. For him, this experience was seen as just one of many experiences building towards a lifetime profession. He was not trying to make any decisions. Interestingly, although he was going through the doctoral transition, all of his dream drawings referred to his experiences of leaving his homeland of Morocco and moving to Germany. For example, in the dream drawing in Figure 6.3, he is with his family in a German city, and they are trying to find a bank. They go from one place to another feeling very confused until they finally reach a bank.

This person's experience demonstrates that what dominates one's dreams are the most important transitions one is undergoing, even if the workshop theme ostensibly says otherwise. And very often, this is a transition that the dreamer did not realise was so dominant in his or her life, as was the case above. It also demonstrates that one very powerful life change is changing cultures, as was the case for a member in the London group who had moved there from Ireland (see Chapter 7). Moving countries and moving cultures are sources of some very rich and important dream material. In any case, this opportunity to review enabled, as Fran in the London group notes, 'all of us to witness ... a story of personal and life transition for each'.

Chapter 7

Extended integration of Social Dream-Drawing learning

In Chapter 6, in which I described the final review session, I detailed various ways in which Social Dream-Drawing (SDD) participants can integrate their learnings on an individual level. This chapter focuses on the broader goal of integrating learning as a group. Because each session focuses on individual dreams, what is often lost is the collective experience and collective insight related to the particular theme of the series of workshops.

When a group is assigned an activity to do together, they have the opportunity to broaden their insights into the predominating themes. Thus they are able to explore such questions as What have we learnt as a group about retirement and the issues associated with it? What are the special challenges of doing a doctorate? What are the most common roadblocks to becoming a researcher?

While this method focuses on individual dream drawings, in a paradoxical way, the group is the engine of learning. Individual learning would not take place without group participation. All participants benefit from the associations offered by other members and by discussions with them, and from articulating and sharing dream experiences with others. One participant's associations spark further associations in others. This takes place constantly. All follow-up events continue to benefit from the group's wisdom, with the goal of increasing learning that can be taken back home and to the workplace.

As described in depth in Chapter 6, one design idea I have used for fuelling this collective learning is the construction of a collective timeline, which I recommend in particular for groups who meet multiple times. In such an exercise, participants are asked to fill in important events that have taken place in their personal lives, their professional lives and in the world at large during the course of the workshop. They each record their data on a large piece of paper. As each person makes an entry, others become stimulated to record similar events or experiences. As such, I have found this to be an excellent way to capture the overall experience of the workshops.

There are various ways to prepare participants for such an exercise. As described in the last chapter, they could be asked first to create individual timelines, using the resources of transcripts or a retrospective viewing of all

DOI: 10.4324/9780429275647-8

the dream drawings. Their entries on the collective timeline are then drawn from these personal timelines. In entering their individual data at the same time as the others, they immediately note the differences and similarities.

Another approach is to ask participants to create a personal timeline at home and to bring it to the next session. This has the advantage of time (saving the need for a workshop session to create individual timelines) and the disadvantage of cutting short individual learnings.

In any case, before data can be entered on a collective timeline, participants must have the time and space to think about the details, consult their diaries and make their choices. Very often, not all information in the personal timeline is entered on the collective one. As with the decision to choose which dream drawing you want to bring to a workshop, participants share only the personal data they wish to share with the others.

However this assignment is approached, what is significant is that the participants are creating a collective document. Up until now, all of their drawings have been individual; this is the first group drawing.

I introduced this activity to the London research group by first asking them to try to recall what had been going on their lives on a personal level and a professional level during the course of our workshop. (Sometimes, consulting one's diary is quite helpful in this instance.) I also asked them to see if they could recall the major world events that took place during that time, especially those that had a direct effect on them. A good example of that is the strike of public workers in London that forced members of this group to decide on which side of the fence they would stand (as described later in this chapter).

I encouraged them as well to consider events that took place slightly before we started the workshops. For example, we learnt that one participant had just been tested for cancer and, when the group began, was still awaiting the results.

In order to differentiate their data, each participant used a different coloured marker to make his or her entries on the group timeline.

In the process of entering data on the group timeline, there are moments of individual thought, clarifying discussion and writing (as seen in Figure 7.1).

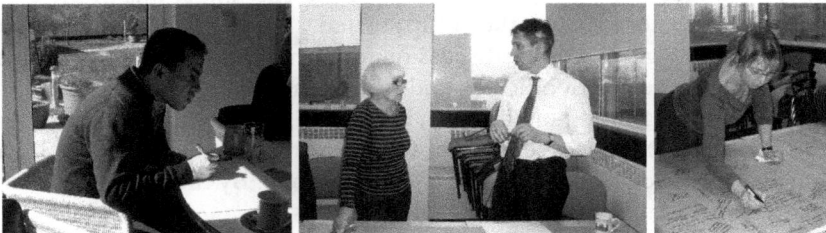

Figure 7.1 Creating the group timeline

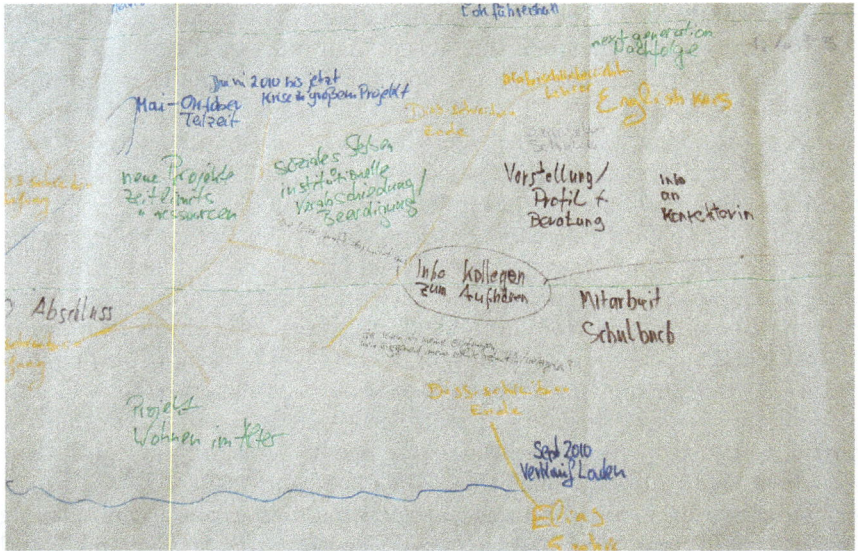

Figure 7.2 Segment of German timeline

Once the entire chart is completed, participants then have a chance to look at the full picture, which is chockful of detail. As an example of this, Figure 7.2 shows a section of the timeline created by the German research group. Note that entries are in different colours for different participants.

Discussion following creation of the timeline

With both groups that created a timeline in this way, the discussion following this activity centred not surprisingly on the key themes experienced by the participants themselves.

I have mentioned earlier how, in the German group of four participants, three were facing decisions about retirement from long-term work in city administration, elementary school administration and university teaching. The fourth, much younger participant, and the only male, was in the early stages of his doctorate when the group started.

For the retiring women, the discussion following the creation of the timeline focused on separation, losses and transformation. As one of them put it: 'It was the beginning of the end'. It seemed as if the experience of the workshop had served as a 'container for the restructuring of their lives', as described by my colleague who observed the group. By the end of our work together, all had made their retirement decisions.

But there were also ideas of a new beginning, of succession, heritage and the next generation (as represented by the fourth group member, perhaps).

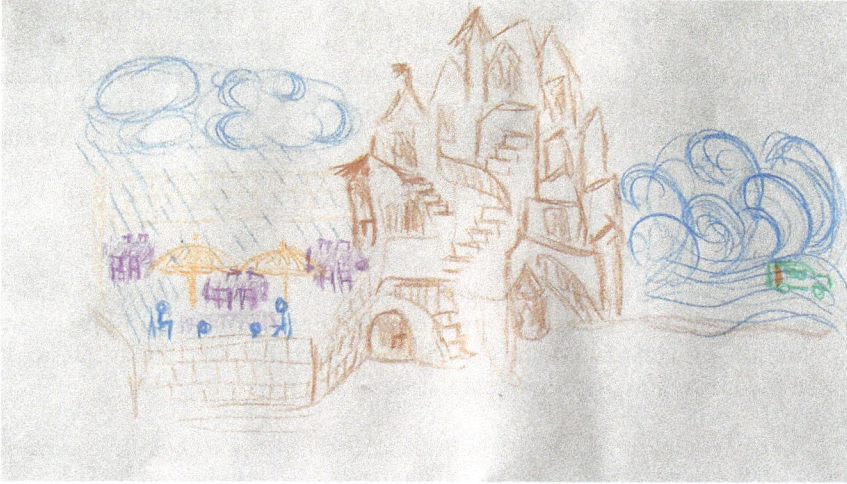

Figure 7.3 The castle

There was mention of the moral dilemma of choosing whether to rescue a very old person or a very young one. Who do you rescue? Both are alive, but the older one has only a short time to live and the younger one a lot longer.

For these women, who were on their way to leaving institutions to which they had dedicated their professional lives, there were not many good feelings about the new. It was difficult for them to imagine creating something fresh. They were in the process of mourning what they were soon planning to leave. Perhaps one strong representation of this were the many dream drawings of large buildings, typical of city administrations, universities and schools. These buildings had offered protection and security, as suggested by the dream drawing in Figure 7.3.

The brick building and the tower appearing in dream drawings of a member of this group are other examples (see Chapters 1 and 6).

The discussions and the learnings by the London group related to the timeline were similar to those of the German research group. In preparation for this work, I offered the London group a maxim for the session, which was: 'The integration of our internal work here and our outside work'. By this, I meant to set the stage for these participants to relate their work with their dream drawings (and the dream drawings of the others) to the context of the wider world, particularly the world of work.

Public sector cutbacks

As it turned out, the workshops in London took place from 2010 to 2011 during a time of extreme budget cutbacks relating to the 2008 economic crisis. These cutbacks had a huge effect on three of the participants, who were working in the public sector at the time. Among other challenges, there were the questions of making people redundant and whether or not to cross picket lines. These dilemmas, which were directly related to our theme of 'What do I risk in my work?', were discussed at length in the review session.

One participant had been particularly troubled by what he was forced to do. As he put it:

> ... in terms of austerity, how that diminishes resources which affects schools, which affects my work role. I've had to make staff redundant and the impact of that on people's families really [was difficult]. I made someone redundant again just before Christmas.

Another participant spoke at length about her dilemma regarding a trade union strike in her workplace. Here is her extended statement:

> We had a very big public sector strike ... in the UK about ten days ago. And it's one of the biggest ones for quite a long time. And I'm working as a contractor, so I'm not a public sector employee but I'm working in the public sector. And I was intending to work and on the night before [the] strike, I and about ten colleagues – actually about twenty colleagues – were going out for dinner .... and we had a young trainee near us .... She must have been about twenty-one and she hadn't decided whether she was going to strike or not. And so she was asking us why we weren't striking, because there was a pile of us there. And what we got into in the dialogue was that we were not striking in order to let other people strike, so that we were holding the duty of care to our service users, because it's vulnerable people that we look after. So in our minds, we had reconciled ourselves that we could come in to let others strike. And so she thought that was interesting; she was just quizzing us a little bit about it. And then in the conversation I was thinking how could I represent that as I cross the picket line, because I will have to cross the picket line. And actually I would like to have a dialogue with the picket line as I cross it. And in the discussion – and it was somebody else's idea; it wasn't mine – one of my colleagues said, 'You know what I hadn't thought about this before, but I'm going to donate my day's pay to the Welfare Fund.' And I thought, what a fantastic idea. So as I came in and as I crossed the picket line, I stopped and talked to the picket line, and all the shop stewards were there and so on. And I said, 'You know what, I'm not an employee, I'm a contractor, but I totally agree with what you're doing, this is why I'm coming in, but I'm going to give you my pay.' So I ended up feeling fantastic; they thought I was great for the moment.

But I wouldn't have got[ten] myself into that position had I not been challenged by a youngster who was trying to question my ethics....So it felt quite a pivotal moment really, kind of discovering something about my own ethics being challenged by the next generation if you like, who are inheriting the economic difficulties that we've helped to create and that I've helped to create no doubt .... But actually my kind of professional journey has been about clarifying my ethics, I think, in relation to others.

In terms of the theme of this workshop, 'What do I risk in my work?', both of these participants had taken great risks in terms of who they were and how they would take their public sector roles forward under the current difficult circumstances. In the SDD workshop, they were able to have a conversation about these dilemmas in a safe setting.

What followed these exchanges was the fascinating observation that in the act of filling in the events on the group timeline, the participants had discovered that there were major connections between them and between their dream drawings.

Here, for example, are two dream drawings from two different members of this group, shown in Figure 7.4. They both depict journeys, travelling and going from one place to another. One is of a person walking (Figure 7.4a) and the other depicts boats on a river (Figure 7.4b). They represent the fact that these participants are in some sort of transition.

Another commonality is the lack of colour in these drawings and their relatively primitive depictions.

As one participant put it:

> ... we actually...blended somehow .... the pictures ... feel more connected now, in my mind anyway .... it could have been one dream ... I'm struck by this because actually they're not in different blocks, they're kind of integrated and sort of filled in gaps between.

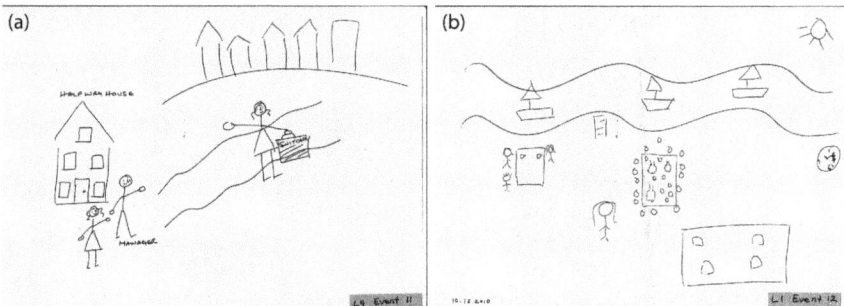

Figure 7.4 Person walking (a) and boats moving (b)

This activity, in fact, brought together four people who, during the course of the workshop, had not had the opportunity earlier to really explore their connections with each other. Another commented:

> Actually I felt when you asked the question about what was happening in the world, I felt that I didn't write an awful lot down here. Because when I started to do that, what was written was a sense of other people allowing to speak for you in a way that I didn't feel like my voice was being taken away. But actually there was no need to say it a second time.

As a final comment, one participant noted, 'It's quite fascinating in the last exercise when you see how it interconnected'.

As in the German group, there was one participant in the London group who had moved countries during the span of the workshop series. Again, her dream drawings and her experience of moving dominated her work with the group. For example, here is one of her dream drawings (Figure 7.5), which dramatises her returning to her house in her native Ireland, only to find it occupied by renters and no longer her home.

She describes how the dream represented her experience at the time:

> I think it was to do with going back and renting out my house and arriving at the house and it not being my house, and not having a sense of

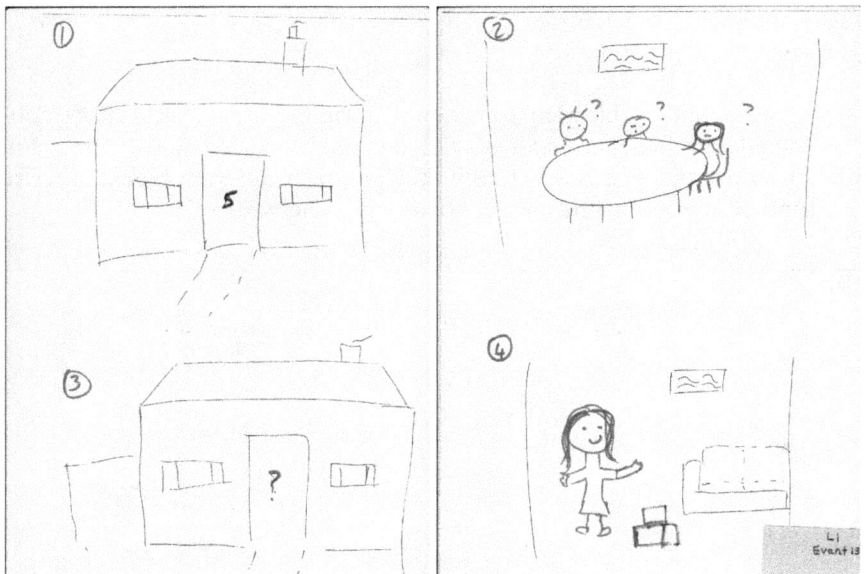

Figure 7.5 Where is home?

where I belonged. Yeah, so I think there was that time, certainly at the end of last year and earlier this year of just not knowing, of knowing where I wanted to be, but not knowing whether I would be able to make it.

Despite this uncertainty, however, she finds herself now 'very settled and very happy professionally and personally in London'. She continues:

> I'm just conscious that when we started in October of last year I had no idea of where I was going to be. And though I wanted to stay in London it might have been not possible financially ....
>
> It's not been easy by any manner or means, but ... it's allowed me to stay in London and allowed me to settle in London ... being settled and asking for help and being able to access help. And being able to take up help when it's offered as well, whereas before there might have been a bit of shield of 'Don't come near me!'
>
> So, yeah, that's been my year ... [I]t's odd to think that ... a lot of the stuff that has happened in the last twelve months, in a kind of global perspective, has been so horrendous. And listening to other Irish people who have come to the UK more recently or are staying in Ireland and having such miserable lives, my life seems to be in complete contrast to that.

For this participant, as with a German participant who had moved from Morocco, as mentioned in Chapter 6, the group experience helped her make the transition, and she was able to express this to everyone in a very satisfying way.

The big picture

Whenever one holds a series of workshops over time, one must keep in mind how important it ultimately may be for the participants to be given the opportunity to put into words what this experience has meant to them and to place this experience in the context of their individual life experience.

Asking these participants to create these timelines has been one avenue towards achieving this goal. It has the great advantage of being another assignment involving drawing, which echoes the act of dream drawing. However, there are many other possible activities in a review session. For example, participants could be asked to bring photographs to this last session from their lives that represent this time of transition.[1] Or they could be asked to bring poems that they have written or that have inspired them during this time.[2]

For some participants, the review session is the opportunity to express, in a major way, the deep importance of the SDD workshop experience. For example, one participant explained:

> ... I have a sense there's some connection, obviously maybe this group contained me in a way that I didn't realise that it was containing me. Or

the expectation perhaps that I was going to go back in September and talk about it. So I suppose the knowing that we would meet again is some form of a connection, containment as well, even if the time frames, the time spans are quite large. I suppose after today when we do formerly finish, there won't be that expectation that we'll come back here.

As with all such intense workshop experiences, all involved must cope with the ending. This chapter has described some of the key ways in which one can harvest the intense and meaningful experience and, by helping participants recognise what they have learnt, provide them with insights that they will take back into their ongoing lives, where they will continually be in transition.

Notes

1 Sievers, B. (2013) Thinking organizations through photographs: the Social Photo-Matrix as a method for understanding organizations in depth. In: Susan Long, ed., *Socioanalytic Methods: Discovering the Hidden in Organisations*. London: Karnac, pp. 129–151.
2 Grisoni, L. (2012) Poem houses: an arts based inquiry into making a transitional artefact to explore shifting understandings and new insights in presentational knowing. *Journal of Organizational Aesthetics*. 1 (1).

Chapter 8

The role of facilitator

There are, of course, many tips and suggestions I could offer to anyone who decides to use the Social Dream-Drawing (SDD) method with others. However, the primary guidance I want to offer in this chapter has to do with conducting yourself in each session in such a way that all the participants feel safe and able to work with others and learn.

As will be clear by now, sharing dream material can make people feel vulnerable. It is, after all, out of one's conscious control. It is not edited by our ego. It has the power to reveal what we would often prefer not to know ourselves, much less share with others. And because of this, even the most sophisticated participants may approach this sort of workshop with a degree of anxiety. For example, Fran, in the London group, explained:

> I think I felt more anxiety at the beginning in that I didn't know in prac-
> tice how ... we're going to negotiate amongst ourselves and with you ...
> the disclosure of quite potentially intimate struggles .... It was clear to
> me that I was putting personal stuff out for discussion .... [and] part of
> the contract ... is that you open yourself up to a bit of discussion about
> your dream.
>
>   So just a little bit of anxiety about ... what if somebody says some-
> thing I don't like, or if they want to say something that I think some-
> body else won't like, or all that kind of stuff. So just a bit of discomfort
> I think anticipating what that might mean .... I understood that was
> part of the contract ... but equally I had every right to limit how much
> I disclosed if it was too uncomfortable. So I didn't feel coerced in any
> way, but I just felt a bit wary.

I think this participant puts it very well.

Since this method is relatively new and involves the very private material of personal dreams, I try to frame it from the beginning not only as a fairly straightforward method but also as a way of learning rather than burrowing into one's deeper persona. I think this helps people feel more relaxed as well. From the beginning of each session, I talk about how SDD might be used in

DOI: 10.4324/9780429275647-9

other contexts in order to make it clear that this is not a therapeutic intervention. As Fran noted, in the 'scene setting' that I had done, she was reassured by the fact that SDD was 'quite a light intervention – well, a reflective intervention – but actually you don't want people to delve into their deep psychic unconscious too much'.

Many participants have commented that the method of SDD is actually quite simple. One follows a set of clear steps and isn't burdened by the need to understand sophisticated theoretical concepts in order to participate in or to facilitate the process. In particular, those participants who would, in fact, go on to use this method themselves commented that they all could imagine doing it with others, even while they were taking part in the workshop. (Actually, one London participant and one Russian participant did exactly that!)

As London participant, Fran put it: 'It's an accessible methodology … that doesn't feel too frightening, it's not so highly complicated that you have to do [a] two-year course to understand it'.

Or, as Frederick noted,

> …. it's quite a modest intervention with…lots and lots of potential. But I think the modesty is so important because what it helped me do is think, 'Oh I could do that.'

At the same time, however, the facilitation of this modest method involves an element of sophistication. As two London participants commented:

> …. there's something about the method which is modest, but that's not to say that your…delivery wasn't sophisticated, because I think it was very sophisticated.
> But I guess what I'm tapping into was that there was something about the way you … did the work, which was light and playful as well as thought provoking and deep.

So, given this view that the method itself (as described in Chapter 5 of this book) is relatively modest, what are the ingredients of the sophisticated facilitation that participants have noted?

Clarity of purpose – no hidden agendas

There may certainly be many reasons for proposing an SDD workshop to potential participants. When I was undertaking my doctoral work, I told invitees that each workshop was part of my research. Last year, I offered it to a couple of my local colleagues who had just retired as a means of supporting them during their transition from full-time careers. And in the corona months of 2020 and 2021, I offered it to experienced consultants as a way to help them understand how this method would work online.

Embedded in the question of purpose is the question of what I or anyone else who participates will do with the data. The online group knew that our work would be the basis for a chapter in this book (see Chapter 9). The doctoral research groups all knew that our work would form the basis for my doctoral studies and would very likely appear in my dissertation and other publications.

For these two groups, I asked each person to sign a consent form, giving me permission to use the data in publications. Despite this, I always checked back with them every time I used their material to ensure I still had their permission. I found this to be especially important when it came to sharing their dream drawings because of their deeply personal nature. For other groups, purely verbal consent was sufficient. And included in all forms of confidentiality agreements – whether written or verbal – is the agreement by all attending not to share the names of participants with others outside the group.

I would say this act of being completely honest about the purpose of the group and the careful efforts to assure confidentiality are examples of behaviours that most participants wouldn't particularly think about. It is only once the work begins that these reassurances create feelings of trust.

Here, for example, are the comments from one London participant:

> And I think that the way that you introduced it as well at the beginning as – although I can't remember exactly what you said, Rose – but I had a sense that this is an investigation, it wasn't that you were trying to force a view on anybody. You weren't a snake … salesman trying to sell something, but you were investigating something and you were going to make interpretations based on the data that you found. So I think that felt reassuring at the beginning as well …. I had a sense of we were here to investigate this together, and I thought that's interesting …. But I had a sense that there was an enjoyment about this joint endeavour of investigating something. And I thought, 'Oh this could be healing.'

Keep your act together from beginning to end

In all aspects of organising and undertaking this workshop, be sure to have your act together. Perhaps this point will seem completely obvious, but I am including it because I have so often witnessed the consequences of a lack of preparation or unclear boundaries or unexplained changes in my own working life.

By this, I mean show up on time. Answer emails in a timely fashion. Be consistent. Prepare in advance. Follow the schedule. Don't disappear.

These are all obvious behaviours of any good professional, but bear in mind we're talking now about facilitating a workshop where participants can feel quite vulnerable and unsafe. They rely on the facilitator not only for expertise but for reliability and safety. And if the facilitator falters, the workshop fails. I have described such a failure in Chapter 5.

Allow the space for reflection and integration

SDD workshops, while they are scheduled in minutes and hours, are not completely action-packed. The material that arises in associations and drawings can take a while to be absorbed. Very often, participants and facilitators need to think and reflect. Just be. And the facilitator needs to sense this and respect this.

So often, the dream material and the drawings contain layers of meaning. One doesn't immediately 'get' all there is. And also, quite often, those comments that arise after a bit of reflection are of a much deeper character. Often they are comments relating to the theme. In a sense, there is first a phase of immediate reaction to the drawings (colours, shapes, directions, etc.). There then often follows a generally relaxed (and frequently fun) period of associations and ideas. And then, quite often, this reflective time.

As a facilitator, it is not easy to judge this. When do I just wait and when do I move on? The urge is to step in. But it is a skill that can be learnt over time. You will gradually sense and trust the delicate timing of this.

This skill is reflected in the following comment by my London co-facilitator Laura:

> But I also think it's the pace and staying with the experience. I think Rose has got a very light and very gentle but firm way of letting people get to the point. So it's really slowing down a bit like a film, and I think that is quite crucial ... to the methodology. I also had to monitor myself because sometimes I'm faster, and I think to actually slow down allows for a very different way of thinking. A bit like in a film, when you see it in a movie going much slower and staying with it. And not over-interpreting as well ....

And also by London participant Louise:

> I think it was the timing around space for me [that] felt quite important and maximising what potentially could be pulled from the drawings and the dreams. It didn't feel like it was rushed at all, sitting with that space.

In a sense, a facilitator should keep to the timetable, but between those boundaries, he should be sensitive to the need for space and reflection.

Respect

Yes, I know this is another obvious point, but I want to include it because this word came up so often in my follow-up research interviews, and it was only in hindsight that I realised how important this concept was for the participants and what I did that was experienced as respectful.

What was cited over and over again was that I showed respect by keeping to the schedule (starting and ending on time, for example). Here, for example, are Fran's comments about this:

> And I think it dissipated because the conversations were respective [respectful] of each other and the boundaries, the time boundaries and the room boundaries and all that were held appropriately and provided containment. So the containment was there but the behaviours were also thoughtful and respectful of everybody in the room.

There are ways of holding time boundaries that are experienced as respectful, and there are ways of holding them that seem autocratic and illogical; for example, by ending a session in the middle of someone's sentence.

Often keeping to the schedule is seen as providing containment, i.e. safety, so that people can work together. But what I learnt is that it is also a way of me, as facilitator, saying to participants: 'Look, I respect your time table, your commitments, and your pressures, and I am not going to abuse them by showing up late or allowing the workshop to go on longer than agreed'.

Anything that has to be changed has to be negotiated. For example, at the end of the review session with the German group, I asked if we could collectively negotiate an extra 15 minutes at the end, in order to fully say our goodbyes.

I have also noticed that ending early is a kind of gift. People are extremely grateful. It is not that the workshop has not been a good experience, but it's only one small part of their very busy lives.

How to hold and keep to time boundaries is a skill one learns over time. Sometimes, especially when there is extensive talking or when there is, perhaps, no talking, it helps to announce that we have five minutes left. Sometimes I do this by picking up on one of the last words said by a participant and using it in a sentence to communicate that we are at the end of the session. For example, in an online group, one last association was to the end of an era of history (i.e. Second World War), which I followed with the comment that we are now at the end of our association era. And sometimes, when it is clear that all has been said, I just end a phase early. This works particularly well when the next phase is a small break. People are always grateful for longer breaks!

One last observation about respect involves the role of humour in this work. Because dream drawings often contain such amazing and unexpected images, there is often a lot of laughing and fooling around during the free-association periods. Vince and Broussine have made the point that working with drawings helps to 'contain the playful as well as the serious'.[1] This is just a natural part of the work. But one has to be careful with this. Dream drawers can be especially sensitive to the playful comments of others, as I have described earlier in Chapter 3. I think it's a safe bet always to keep in mind that while laughter and fun are intrinsic to this method, this should never be at the expense of another. As Frederick from the London group put it: 'You were inviting us to be playful, but you weren't toying with us'.

Feel safe ... not the source of turbulence

Any workshop that delves into the deeper recesses of our unconscious is bound to stimulate uncomfortable feelings. When these feelings arise in a gradual fashion, when they can be spoken about, when they are shared by others in a group situation, tolerable doses of revelation can be integrated ... step by step. This workshop is, after all, not designed as a therapeutic intervention. That said, however, it very often has a therapeutic impact.

One key characteristic of such an experience is that there is sufficient structure and sufficient time for participants to 'take in' these uncomfortable feelings and, before the end of the day, begin to integrate them. Otherwise, one leaves the safety and security of the workshop environment feeling overwhelmed and more unsettled than when it began. The goal is for that not to happen.

By choosing which dream drawing to bring or by choosing not to bring any dream drawing at all, participants self-manage their exposure. Some participants take more risks than others. Some put more effort into their drawings than others. Some bring dream drawings with very private material included. The longer a workshop lasts over time, generally, the more risky the material brought to the group. This is a sign that people feel safe enough to share.

In response to a comment that the workshop creates turbulence, London participant Louise put it this way:

> I don't see it like that. Because I think what you get from bringing the drawings here is the opportunity to discuss what's currently going on in your mind, in a way you probably wouldn't do. So I think you may bring in your own turbulence. But in fact on talking and focusing on that on the drawings you can bring it out more, and it gives you something more to think about than you would have got if you hadn't gone through that process.

As another participant put it: 'It's not going to leave you flapping in the wind with it'.

Ethical awareness

I assume that anyone taking the time to read this book and, particularly, to read this chapter is already quite aware of the various ethical issues surrounding this sort of workshop. But I will just highlight a few that I consider especially relevant to this work.

I have always found ethical considerations to be one of the last issues mentioned when one organises a workshop. I am guilty of that myself. It's as if, 'Oh, by the way, do you agree, we will keep this confidential among ourselves?' As if everybody assumes the same thing and it isn't even worth mentioning.

But that actually isn't always so. In fact, I think that the mere act of prioritising ethics and voicing this directly is already about behaving in an ethical way. It is communicating to participants that ethics are important to 'me', the facilitator and that, therefore they are going to be important to all of us.

I think of ethical issues in relation both to what happens during the face-to-face (or Zoom-to-Zoom) time and to what happens 'outside' of the direct workshop experience. While the workshop is taking place, one behaves ethically by treating all with respect and acceptance. This means being careful never to criticise or exclude anyone from participation. It also involves being sensitive to emotional overload and giving every participant the right to exit the group at any point in the process.

Ethical considerations 'outside' the main event primarily concern confidentiality. As mentioned earlier, having published so many articles on this method, even if they have previously agreed, I ask participants once more to give me permission to use whatever material we generate for my publications. Normally participants take this request quite lightly as if it is obvious. Some participants of long standing have given me life-long permission to use their drawings. Nevertheless, whenever I publish a piece that includes someone's dream drawing, I check in advance if it ok. This is largely because of the drawings, which can be instantly recognisable by the drawer and by his or her fellow participants. And in being recognised in this way, the drawings can immediately bring back the emotional content of the dream.

Pairing with other professionals

Over the course of the many years that I have facilitated SDD workshops, I have invited colleagues to work with me in various roles, mostly to support and to help me develop the method. Sometimes these helpers remain in the background, as was the case with my German supervisor, with whom I met regularly during my doctoral studies. Sometimes, they are observers who do not participate but who offer insight and guidance. Sometimes these colleagues serve as translators, as happened with my colleagues in Chile and Germany. And sometimes, they serve as co-facilitators.

Similar to the decision to bring a colleague into a client organisation, the choice of who to invite to attend a workshop as a fellow facilitator or observer involves a sense of trust in the other person. The great advantage of a co-facilitator is that this lessens the overall burden of leading the entire workshop. (This was a choice I made when I ran a two-day workshop in Oxford, for example.)

In the case of one online workshop, I invited a younger colleague to manage all the Zoom details so that I could lead and fully participate in the workshop. In order to reassure the participants that this person was a part of the workshop and would follow all ethical agreements and assumptions, we presented ourselves as a working partnership. He introduced himself at the beginning of each session and dealt with all participants by email.

One last category is those professionals or colleagues who have asked me to run SDD workshops with their own groups. In some cases, these have been groups of doctoral students. In another instance, it was a group of alumni from a master's programme. Another was at the invitation of a professional organisation, as part of their professional development programme. Very often, these colleagues manage all the organisational details, which is a relief for me. And normally, this person participates just like any other participant, but without bringing a dream drawing.

Being mindful of the leader's influence and status

Lastly, I want to mention an aspect of group dynamics and authority. In any SDD workshop, there is a hierarchy, both formal and informal. As the facilitator, I generally have the most authority and, therefore, the most responsibility. Other colleagues – who have been brought in to host, to partner, to translate or to observe – come next. And among the participants, there is often a hierarchy as well (student and teacher, boss and employee, higher position in sponsoring organisation vis a vis a lower position, or informal leaders within a peer group). These hierarchical differences are often sensed but never talked about. And the facilitator cannot always know about them.

All the facilitator can be sensitive to is his or her own hierarchical status. The facilitator is the expert in this method, and thus any comment the facilitator makes in relation to a dream drawing or anything else carries more weight than those of the others. That is why, for example, I never make the first association to a drawing or a comment on the theme (see Step 4 in Chapter 5). I know from experience that if I do, participants, in the desire to perform well, will follow with similar thinking. And, after all, the goal is creative and original thinking by all present.

Sometimes someone in authority can make a comment that is taken as a criticism, as took place in a London group, where my host colleague was the doctoral examiner of three of the participants. My colleague remarked that a particular drawing (of one of the doctoral students) was 'childlike'. As it turned out, this student took this comment as relating not only to her drawing but to her role as a doctoral student. This was an issue already present in the relationship before the workshop began. And this incident affected another member of the group who said:

> But the stand-out memory in some ways is that the second session where I did present a drawing and somebody said, 'Oh, that's quite childlike.' I thought, 'hmm', it felt a bit like 'oh, excuse me!' And I think a similar comment was made about Fran's drawings as well at one point. In fact I think it might have been made in the very first session .... And I remember thinking when it was first said about Fran, 'Oh I didn't realise that our actual drawing skills were going to be under scrutiny so to speak.'

As a former doctoral student myself, I know very well how sensitive one can be to criticism offered by one's doctoral supervisor. This is just an example of why it is important to be sensitive to the dynamics in the organisation where one is offering this workshop.

There are great advantages to working with colleagues whom you trust, whether in the role of observer, workshop host, Zoom host or co-facilitator. In debriefing the sessions together, you benefit from their insights and expertise regarding the design and conduct of the workshop. With their support, you innovate on the method. And any time an esteemed colleague accepts an invitation to work with you, it is a confirmation that the work has value.

Online facilitation

There is no doubt that the role of facilitation and the capacity of the facilitator are affected when an SDD workshop takes place online. As facilitator, you no longer have the visual cues that come from being face to face and working together. You are no longer able to sit next to the presenter of each drawing in order to support him or her. You are no longer able to physically handle the dream drawing carefully as a sign of respect and help the drawer remove it at a particular point.

In addition, you are now dependent upon a crucial 'other' to manage the Zoom invitations and the various changes in what can be seen and not seen during the course of the workshop (see Chapter 9). So the relationship between the facilitator and the Zoom manager (who is often on the other side of the world) is crucial to a smooth and undisturbed experience.

All of these points and more will be explored in Chapter 9: Coronavirus and working online.

The heart of good SDD practice

SDD, as a method, has been gradually developed and tested by myself through many iterations over a number of years. I believe, in and of itself, it has integrity and logic. There are no major secrets about this method, what the steps are or who can benefit most from it. In the invitation to take part, the method itself should be clearly described. What makes for its effectiveness is the way it is managed and facilitated. And each facilitator of this method will bring his or her own special capacities.

As articulated by management professor Robert French in his description of a good classroom learning space, the method has

> ... both a *paternal* and *maternal* dimension. The paternal relates to the systemic, to the establishment and maintenance of the setting; the maternal to the work (or play) of direct interaction, relationship, and nurture that requires this containing space if it is to thrive.[2]

The goal, as ever, is to achieve what Julie, a participant in the Russian online group, described as 'innovating, indirectly excavating what's lying behind the surfaces of every day rush to produce results and gently revealing deeper barriers and hidden concerns'. I couldn't say it better myself!

Notes

1   Vince, R. and Broussine, M. (1996) Paradox, defense, attachment – Accessing and working with emotions and relations underlying organizational change. *Organization Studies.* 17, p. 17.
2   French, R. (1997) The teacher as container of anxiety: psychoanalysis and the role of teacher. *Journal of Management Education.* 21 (4), p. 488.

Chapter 9

Coronavirus and working online

The scourge of corona in 2020 and 2021 brought challenges and opportunities to all of us professionals. In my case, it challenged me to offer Social Dream-Drawing (SDD) as an online workshop, and this chapter is dedicated to describing how my first workshop was organised and conducted online.

I invited a group of four organisational consultants from Moscow to participate, and, as a group, we decided on the theme 'Who am I online?' This theme captured the dilemmas facing these consultants in their work with their own clients, whom they normally only met face to face, being themselves members of a professional community that is generally sceptical about online work.

The major professional transition facing this group lay in entering the realm of working only online and leaving the world of face-to-face consultation (at least for the time being and, who knows, perhaps much longer). Our goal in selecting this theme was to try to understand how online work would influence our capacity to connect and work effectively with clients.

A face-to-face SDD workshop normally lasts three or four hours, depending on how many dream drawings we work with. Based on my own recent experience, I assumed in advance that a three- or four-hour Zoom workshop would simply be too exhausting and demanding. I, therefore, decided to hold four distinct sessions two weeks apart and a final review session (see Chapter 6) two weeks after that. In each of the four one-hour sessions, we worked with a single dream drawing.

The 'Who am I online?' Zoom SDD workshop

The timing of this workshop was fortuitous because it took place relatively early on in the corona saga, from May 6 to July 7, 2020. This was a period when we were only beginning to take in the reality of this deadly situation and when we were still quite new to constant online interaction.

DOI: 10.4324/9780429275647-10

In each session, we followed the normal design of the workshop (as follows), and the directions in italics at the end of each step refer to what would be shown on the Zoom screen at each step.

- Step 1: The dreamer tells everyone about the dream (3 to 5 minutes). *Show just the dreamer.*
- Step 2: The dreamer shows and explains the drawing (3 to 5 minutes). *Show dreamer and drawing.*
- Step 3: Participants ask clarifying questions of the dream drawer (3 to 5 minutes). *Still showing dreamer and drawing.*
- Step 4: All (including the dreamer and facilitator) offer free associations and amplifications (15 to 20 minutes). *Show only the drawing.*
- Step 5: Dreamer responds to free associations; discussion follows (5 to 10 minutes). *Show everyone; remove drawing.*
- *Everyone stands up, turns around, takes a tiny break ....*
- Step 6: We reflect on the theme (15 to 20 minutes). *Show everyone.*

We were very fortunate to have one member take on the role of Zoom manager, who followed my instructions as to what should be shown on the screen. She was the official Zoom host and reliably moved us around in Zoom land as we went through the steps of the workshop. Her reliability cannot be underestimated, and I will comment more on that later.

Since we now know that when we Zoom, we can be confronted constantly by our own visage (which is exactly the opposite of when we work in person), I wanted to organise the Zoom 'exposure' in such a way that when people participate, they are seen, and when they do not participate, they are able to observe without being seen.

The grounds for these decisions had to do with where we should focus our view. My thought was that gazing at oneself or being gazed at by others would restrict our capacity to free associate (see Step 4 above). In other words, people might feel intimidated or uncomfortable with the visual reactions of others to their free thoughts.

At the same time, however, I wanted the dreamer to be seen by all (Step 1) when she shares the dream so that we may have the benefit of visual clues in working with the drawing. At the stage when everyone begins to share associations to the drawing, I wanted only the drawing to be seen so that our complete attention goes to it.

When we return to the responses of the dreamer to our work, I ask for the drawing to be removed. At that point, all of us can be seen. We are now starting our transition out of the deep primitive dream material back into group life itself.

After the dreamer's comments, we continue to see one another as we discuss the experience and then reflect on the theme of 'Who am I online?'

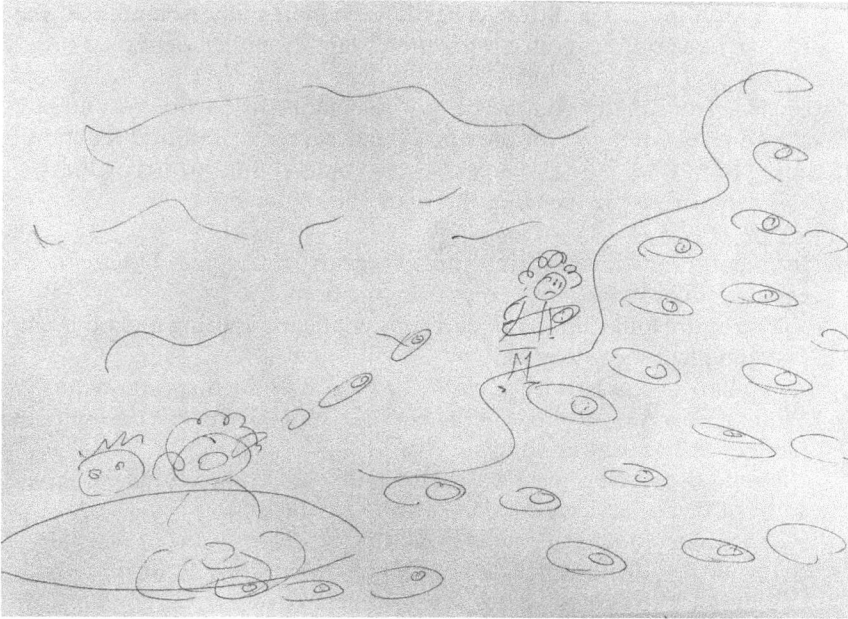

Figure 9.1 Babies in the water

Despite my conviction that setting a theme in advance before participants create their dream drawings mobilises one's internal dream machine to produce dreams relating to this theme, in this case, our theme of working online became only a secondary preoccupation of our group. The primary occupation, which is no surprise, was the coronavirus.

Our very first dream drawing illustrated this, as shown in Figure 9.1.

Petra described her dream this way:

> I had a dream the day after Rose's letter.
>
> I see I am walking along the sea coast, there are many babies on the beach. I lean toward babies to see what happened: are they alive or dead? Many are dead but can I find someone alive? Where [do] they come from? I see the boat far away in the sea. There's a man and a woman in the boat and she gives birth to all these babies – they go out of both her vagina and her mouth.

She described the drawing as follows:

> I did this drawing quick and dirty, just in one minute to fix the dream, it was so emotional I had a feeling I could lose it. I am on the coast ... and hold a baby to understand if it's alive or dead. Babies are on the coast,

the boat is in the sea, I draw a head of the man and a woman, two ways of how babies appear – from her mouth and from her vagina.

It was clear from the beginning of our associations that this was an emotional and tragic dream. Not only had the dreamer a profound reaction to dreaming it, but we, in the group, also responded quite strongly. Our associations soon led to the theme of the virus. They include:

It's a bomb-busting machine and somebody is shooting. Babies are like eggs, or holes in the land, holes from the bombs
    The figure looks upset, no ears, doesn't hear anything and no breath, just complete sorrow, grief
    Woman trying to save a child, to bury a child that would survive. Woman uses two openings in the body to fulfil the frenetic desire to give birth of at least one child to survive
    Obvious association to the virus, and what comes from the mouth, some of these particles are dead and some are alive
    A woman – does she have a live virus?
    Live water, death water (like in fairy tales), live virus, death virus,
    Woman is the virus – it keeps reproducing itself
    Man – just the head – the knowledge. Science, knowledgeable men to give us the answer. But what is here – only round eyes – what [the] bloody hell is happening?
    Woman is trying to decide who to resuscitate or let die

In a sense, this dream and this dream-drawing set the tone for our whole workshop. For each dream drawing, we had very strong associations which led us, almost inevitably, to the virus. There were many themes about loss: Babies in the water, a lost pocketbook, a lost pair of shoes.
    After four sessions, in which we worked with one dream drawing at a time, we held a review session (see Chapter 6) and, looking at the array of four drawings (see Figure 9.2), reflected on our experience and our learnings from our work together.
    In this reflection, many themes were touched upon.
    One had to do with life cycles, as in this comment from the transcript:

I'm connecting all of them in the sequence; just you approach the water in the first one and then you get drawn in and completely immersed: everything is immersed in water. And then the third one with tram, you look for a vehicle to escape from this and then you see this plane's aircrafts escaping.
    I can turn to it as if from a lot of babies in the first picture to a lot of machines in the last picture.

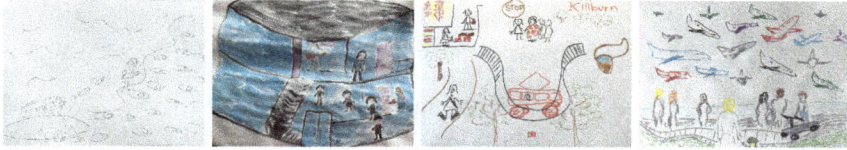

Figure 9.2 'Who am I online?' dream drawings

But then it kind of rebalances back just the fantasy if we go clockwise and then it's ... a never ending spiral and people and the babies being born again and we go through this cycle again.

Another major theme, naturally related to the pandemic, was loss. For example:

And also in general, I have this feeling. About all pictures. The feeling of loss.

I would add lost and being lost.

And today is positive and less dramatic because that's sort of who we are online and what it is online on going back to the pictures. It is painful. It is something like living with a loss and tolerating this living with the loss. And ... maybe it's kind of a loss that you cannot really completely mourn ... because you face it each time you go on Zoom, ... and each time ... it's not your body with you and not the bodies of other people. And with every meeting, you kind of meet again and again with this loss. It's not me with my body and it's not other participants with their bodies there.

Connected to this overarching theme of loss was the loss of the physical contact that corona has forced us into, leading to contempt and fear of our online existence:

And no matter how hard we try, try to find ourselves ... to find some space in this cyber space and the cyber reality to the end ... which I am scared of: that humanity might lose this game ... to the cyber world. What people might probably be able to do is just to stand and watch. How the human relationships are being ruined. Being erased. Being lost.

Right now, it feels so sad and like a lonely traveller in the universe.

Not only are we forced into a cyber world, but we are also dependent on this world in order to be connected to one another:

Like, what I can do in this situation where I can rely upon this Zoom Big Other? I'm totally reliant on it.

What is behind this dependence? That probably even our thinking capacities might be seriously distraught, particularly because this is a kind of internal experience that, you know, at what moment they can stop seeing me or I can stop seeing them.

I lost Internet. Or the Internet lost me, I don't know ... we lost each other.

One of our sessions had to be cancelled because the internet was not functioning in my neighbourhood. And this disruption resulted in one person not being able to attend the next session.

On the other hand, there was a recognition that working on Zoom brings a kind of intimacy. As Gilmore and Warren point out in their article 'Emotion online: Experiences of teaching in a virtual learning environment',[1] online interaction actually leads to more open exchange and a 'greater emotional connection'. Although, as they point out, we lack the familiar physical clues of in-person contact and all of the physical signals of authority and place (i.e. the teacher stands at the front of the room), this is offset by a greater sense of openness and 'emotional expressiveness'[2] in the teaching situation.

While this reality was reflected in a number of different ways in our workshop sessions, there were also expressions of concern about personal exposure on Zoom. This included issues such as what one wears and what background one uses:

I think of exposure in this sense and the need to control, I don't know, as if it were a kind of a dress ... you need to control that it doesn't slip off you all the time. Otherwise, you are naked and you have to ... [be] sure it doesn't fall, it doesn't slip over your shoulder or whatever.

And then one is exposed to oneself in a certain kind of way, which creates a certain strain in the interaction:

Like, you have a lot of mirrors which we don't have in ordinary life. I look at myself [and] see myself actually during the whole of this meeting. I don't in ordinary life, I don't look at the mirror, so, so much.

It's very difficult to relax in this mode, it should be very intense.

And not only do we look at ourselves, but the others look at us:

I'm thinking about what intensifies this infantile anxiety, particularly ... what Anya's saying: it's the gaze of the other.

But here in the Zoom, it's a double intensity. It's you looking at me and I looking at myself. And it's so confusing. Back to your, Anya, ideas about borders. The borders are so obscure that they become so opaque they become so mismatched. The borders of the body. Like, like ...

Well. It's ... like, is it me, what I'm seeing this shape and the shape I'm seeing here?

In a very interesting way, then, on Zoom, one is forced to face oneself, to look at oneself. And, over time, as the experience of face-to-face contact fades and Zoom contact increases, the feelings associated with frequent internet contact intensify. As one participant put it:

> Well, in ordinary life, so to say...we don't feel that much alone phys-ically .... So we now have faced quite a long time when we have been physically alone .... This is like the meeting with yourself, one-on-one with yourself and no one else. Normally in usual life, it would be say, once or three, maybe times a week when if you have psychoanalysis, you meet yourself. And it's not really in the very lonely situation. You have someone else sitting there to rescue you if something goes wrong. But this meeting one-on-one with yourself occurs, well, quite occasionally. And now we've been to it quite a long period of time when we have this internal look at ourselves, glance or reflective glance or the Zooming glance, trying to figure out, look at yourself, what you are doing, what you're saying almost all the time! .... What is terrifying is this looking at myself all the time – even though I try to look at you, by the side of you, I can see myself. I just keep doing this, yes, I cannot stop doing this.

A valuable experience

Despite the sense of disembodiment, strain and exposure brought on by working on Zoom, the method of SDD really did seem to work extremely well online. The great advantage of this method – that it is about the visual – suits it to online work. But in addition to that, the drawings themselves function as a kind of connecting object.

Keeping in mind that the drawings are expressions of the body (see Chapter 2), working with them somehow compensates for the absence of the physical body in online work. As 'the first sensation of the dream' (to quote workshop participant Petra), the drawings visually convey the phys-ical aspects of the dreams themselves, which one can immediately relate to online. And this helps the participants connect with one another. As one participant said:

> ... most definitely, there is the space with less anxiety to connect with a drawing of a person and thus connecting with a drawing, you are ... connected with a person.

One participant described the dream drawings as 'artefacts' of our experi-ence together. Each has her own tangible souvenir of our online experience.

These drawings can easily be photographed and displayed. Online dream drawers made vivid use of colour and detail and, in all cases, provided very rich material for our associations and thoughts.

The critical role of Zoom manager

As the facilitator of this workshop, one question I kept asking myself is: 'How do I facilitate this in a way that participants feel safe enough to work?' When we meet face to face, I am able to sit next to the dream drawer, for example, and use endless physical touches and nods and eye contact to communicate safety. But Zoom is different.

A key element to this sense of safety is how the mechanics of Zoom are managed. In our case, we were very, very lucky. One of our participants took this role and was able to fully participate as well. We were all grateful to her for how she managed it. No one felt at any point excluded or disregarded, which can quickly become the case with mismanaged technology.

This exchange captures our gratitude to our Zoom manager and co-participant:

> And I want to thank you … for bringing us and being so, so reliable, so always on the spot.
> So like your picture. Like a tram in my picture. Yeah.
> The most sturdy of the most secure place I can rely upon. Thank you, Anya.
> We depend on her.
> Exactly.

The reliability of the Zoom manager and the careful and caring way this person took this role served as an important balance to the feelings of vulnerability and dependency on the internet.

For anyone seeking to run an online SDD workshop, therefore, I strongly recommend asking someone else to handle the technical role so that you can concentrate solely on the workshop itself. In another online SDD group that I ran, I invited a colleague to take the role of Zoom manager. He and I worked as a team to conduct the workshop. Our good working relationship enabled me (and us) to focus on the work we were doing.

We also discovered that having an external Zoom manager who is not participating in the workshop ran the risk that the group would experience itself as being observed and perhaps judged by this technical person. Therefore we took many steps to build his relatedness to the participants. For example, he was responsible for all the email contact with them during the course of the program.

Further thoughts and learnings

One participant in another online SDD workshop found this method to work perfectly online. She cited research done on the advantages of working from a familiar setting (i.e. home) and the sense of security and familiarity that brings. Another noted that working from home was much more productive for her. This is also described by Francesca Cardona, an organisational consultant in London, in her 2020 book, *Work Matters,*[3] which was written before the corona crisis began. In it, she mentions two clients whose work with her was actually more productive online than in person and describes virtual consultancy this way:

> In both their situations, it provided a more effective 'consultancy stage'. Both clients were able to feel grounded in their familiar territory. From that 'safe' base, they were able to engage differently with me and overcome some of the barriers of a more conventional space where they felt less connected ... The potential disadvantages of the virtual element and the physical distance are balanced by the connection with a familiar base that might create more possibilities.[4]

This has also been my experience in working for many years with a client who, although she lived quite close to me, always preferred working with me by telephone.[5]

Naturally, there is the problem of the invasiveness of the Zoom method. One participant, for example, always used a green cityscape screen behind her in order to hide her personal space. She likened the glass bowl in her dream drawing (Figure 9.2b) to the Zoom screen, where all can be seen. For her, one is more exposed online.

In the follow-up interviews, another participant noted that as difficult as it was to be confronted with the dream drawings and the issues they raised, this forum was the only one she had where she could truly share her deeper experiences of the virus. It was, for her, a safe and open space where she could deeply experience the terror and sadness she experienced. In all other areas of her life, like the rest of us, she just had to get on with it.

Yet another participant likened the workshop to an 'interesting short journey'. It was like going to the forest, sitting around the fire and sharing some stories. Warm and cosy. She was happy that she did it.

Going forward, I decided to change the structure of these sessions in one particular way. The structure of only doing one dream drawing at a time and then immediately going offline turned out to be quite difficult. Normally, in a face-to-face workshop, we would be together for half a day. Even if we started out with a difficult dream drawing, raising many difficult feelings, the physical connection, the chats during the coffee breaks, and the general experience of being together for a period of time would often mitigate the effects of such an experience. However, that was not the case with our workshop. Therefore, I now add an extra fifteen minutes after the end just to 'chat' and be together informally, as a kind of opportunity to 'des-stress' ourselves (in an informal reflective space).

I think it's important to take into consideration than when one works face to face and has to travel to and from a very deep experience, there is a built-in 'transitional space'[6] in which to reflect and prepare. But with Zoom, it is all about your face without this transitional cushion. We turn immediately to yet another Zoom interaction or just back to what's going on next at home.

For all four participants, this workshop helped them to recognise the kinds of feelings and stresses that they and their clients were experiencing working online. This enabled them to develop their own coping mechanisms (such as using the function of going dark and not seeing their own faces when working or using a background green screen) to manage this work. Having a deeper understanding of their own struggles with this online medium, they find themselves much better prepared to undertake this sort of work with their clients.

Notes

1 Gilmore, S. and Warren, S. (2007) Emotion online: experience of teaching in a virtual learning environment. *Human Relations*. 60 (4), p. 586.
2 Ibid., p. 587.
3 Cardona, F. (2020) *Work Matters: Consulting to Leaders and Organizations in the Tavistock Tradition*. London: Routledge.
4 Ibid., p. 95.
5 Mersky, R. (2006) Organizational role analysis by telephone: the client I met only once. In: Newton, J., Long, S. and Sievers, B., eds. (2006) *Coaching in Depth: The Organizational Role Analysis Approach*. London: Karnac, pp. 113–125.
6 Winnicott, D.W. (1967) The location of cultural experience. *International Journal of Psychoanalysis*. 48, pp. 368–372.

Chapter 10

Other ways of using Social Dream-Drawing

In this book, I have described in detail how to undertake a Social Dream-Drawing (SDD) workshop. This has included descriptions of the various preparatory steps, the step-by-step directions for the method, guidance on facilitation and various post-workshop activities that enhance the learnings. However, there are also ways in which the basic principles underlying this method can be adapted and applied to other situations; for example, I mentioned in the last chapter how the method can be adapted for online work.

The basic principles of SDD are these:

1 Ample time for the dreamer to tell the dream and then show the drawing.
2 A period of free association to the dream, the drawing, and the telling
3 An opportunity for the dream drawer to respond to this experience
4 A general discussion of the experience
5 Reflection on its meaning by the group

While my research and experience first demonstrated that SDD is especially valuable for individuals going through a major transition, it has been used in other situations. As Julie in the Russian group put it, 'I also see it as a useful method of working both individually and at the organisational level, particularly when people face challenges of little known origin which create a high level of anxiety'. In this chapter, I will be sharing four different examples of how colleagues of mine and I myself have adapted the SDD method in the hopes that those interested in SDD will feel free to adapt it to other situations as well.

A method for understanding group dynamics

A colleague has been working for some time online, supervising a group of new organisational coaches. She runs the sessions so that there is first an opportunity for reflecting on individual work (for example, people may share individual consulting dilemmas or questions), which is followed by a period of looking at the group itself, i.e. how the group is

DOI: 10.4324/9780429275647-11

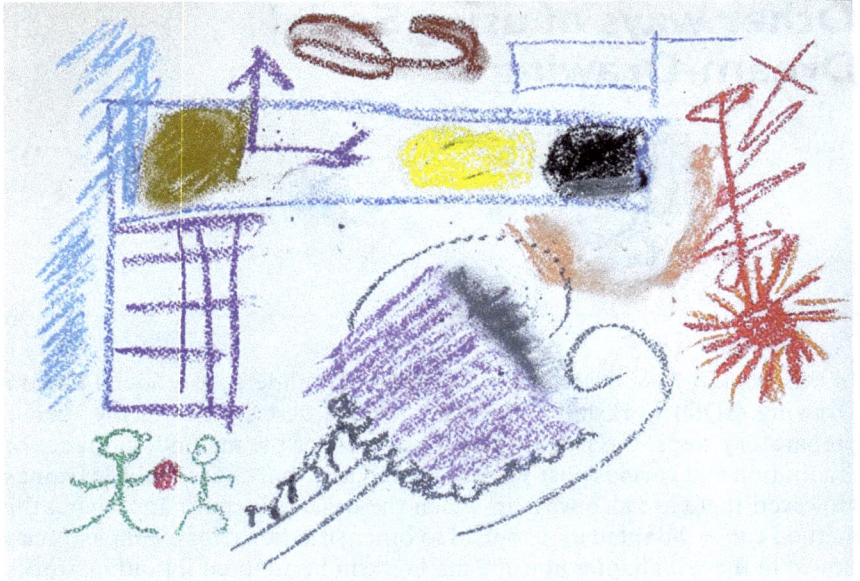

Figure 10.1 Myself as elevator

working together, what conflicts are arising, and what feelings people have about the group.

This colleague had already invited participants to share their dreams in these sessions. She told me, 'I said that if they have a dream and they want to share and they think that it's about our group just ... bring it'.

Sure enough, with this encouragement, a participant brought along a dream drawing (Figure 10.1) to one of these sessions, which they then used to explore the 'situation in the group'. My colleague went on to explain, 'This is a dream [that] came up after our group started'. In other words, something in the group discussions prompted the dreamer to remember this dream, which 'helped us to start a conversation about the group's feelings and expectations'.

She described the dream and drawing as follows:

> The SDD was about an elevator that cannot be controlled – on the one hand the elevator can move in any direction and take a person any-where; on the other hand it was completely unmanageable. This dream took place in the second session of our group and helped us to start a conversation about feelings around uncertainty, which was created by [the] psychodynamic method, COVID situation and a new role [this was a group of newly qualified coaches]. Also, this SDD helped to start [a] conversation about my role: 'Who am I to them?' Me as this elevator who

can move ... anywhere, and this is about 1) my omnipotence and their dependency on me; 2) their loss of control and anxiety; 3) my power over them and anger at me; 4) their high expectations, which I must satisfy.

My colleague made the point that using dream material not only 'helped us to go deeper', but also 'makes the process faster', in the sense that 'we go exactly in the right place' using this method. An experienced supervisor such as my colleague was thus able to use this important material creatively, even with unexperienced trainee coaches.

Another example of the capacity of the method comes from a London colleague who made use of a dream drawing with a group of six health workers that he was supervising once a month. In the course of their work, he invited them to bring dream drawings. He suggested that these illustrations would illuminate the issues they were experiencing in their work roles. In this case, he did not identify a theme in advance. Instead, the work with dream drawings happened like this:

And the reason it came about, Rose, was that someone had had some quite disturbing dreams that they spoke about in a consultancy group. And I invited them and said, 'Well, Rose Mersky did this work which I'm part of and if you would like to give it a go we can do this next session if you'd like to bring [a dream drawing].' And they did – in fact, three people did.

One of the drawings was of a 'city on fire on a hill and a sea full of sharks' ('very powerful imagery'). At first the dream drawer related this dream drawing to her personal situation. But when my colleague asked her, 'What does this mean for our work?' the group very quickly identified the ways in which this dream drawing related both to their own 'separate professional dilemmas' and also served as a paradigm for the organisations themselves in which they worked.

Unfortunately, my colleague could not locate a photo of this drawing, but when reflecting on the experience, he noted:

[T]hey absolutely lapped it up, to be honest. They got a tremendous amount from it ... They were quite astonished about what they got back from it, and just how deeply it related. And there was that sense of astonishment and shock ... My sense with them was that they were absolutely stunned by what they had come up with, really ... Some of the dreams were fantastic, so rich, they were tremendously useful in terms of delivering insight.

It is important to note about these two examples that these colleagues, who had both previously participated in an SDD workshop with me, felt secure enough with dream drawings to spontaneously invite their supervisees to produce one for the group to work with. In the first example, the supervisor invited the participants to bring drawings of dreams that they had had only since the group began.

And in the second example, the person first talked about the dream and then made the drawing on the spot. Normally, as mentioned earlier, I require that dream drawings be done before the group meets because my emphasis is on the individual's experience. But in this case, it was better to have the dreamer draw while she was with the group in order for the group dynamic to be reflected in the material.

An intervention in a group full of intergenerational conflict

As a student in a graduate class called 'Researching the Unconscious', I was invited by our instructor to offer an SDD workshop to the group. We were a class of 6 women, 2 younger students (both in their 20s), one student in her mid-30s, and 3 of us who were over 50 years old. On accepting the invitation to do the workshop, I introduced the concept of SDD to everyone and asked if someone would like to suggest a theme. The youngest suggested the following: 'To what extent does generation play a role in research?'

As it turns out, this theme came to represent a major conflict in the group, which at that point had not yet surfaced.

As part of the requirements for the course, we were all expected to do a small project about the unconscious. At the point at which my workshop took place, a number of students had still not been able to come up with a suitable project to research. The younger participants were particularly at a loss. What was so fascinating is that through this workshop, we were able to identify and explore a key dynamic in this group of six that appeared in retrospect to be hindering the participants from fulfilling the project requirements. In a sense, the dynamics in the group had so overwhelmed the participants that they could not think about a project.

Here is how it happened ...

Two people (the second-youngest participant and the participant in her thirties) each brought dream drawings to the workshop.

Figure 10.2 shows the dream drawing of the participant in her thirties, who went first.

This drawing depicts a very big space, with hospital beds suspended from the ceiling. The dreamer is lying in one of the beds. When her doctor enters, she starts to feel 'uncomfortable' and 'vulnerable'. This doctor is actually the dreamer's therapy client, who is older than the dreamer.

Associations to the dream drawing related to this inter-generational relationship, e.g.: 'inferiority', 'mother and child', 'parent and child' and 'the mother putting you to bed'. Here the doctor is both patient and healer, and

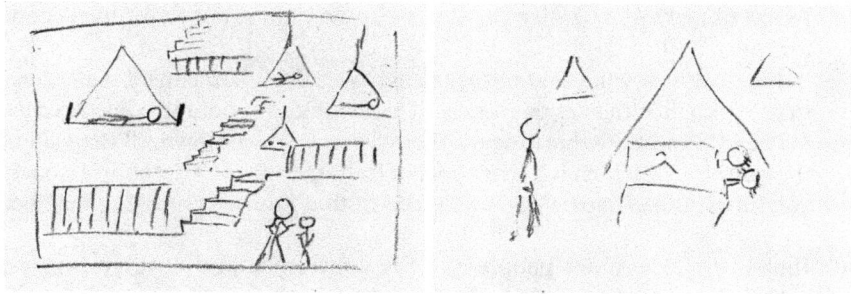

Figure 10.2 Suspended hospital beds

the dreamer is both patient and healer. There is a 'role reversal'. It is 'spooky', 'complicated' and 'awkward'.

The discussion following the free associations helped to crystallise one of the major dynamics in the group, i.e. the generational differences between the two sub-groups, with one person (the dreamer) finding herself in the middle.

As one of 'the oldies' noted, 'We are at the extremes really'. Another noted: 'One of the things you learn as you grow older is that you can survive what you didn't think you can survive'. Another said that it is 'hard to be an older learner'.

Younger participants had their say as well, for example: 'Just because I'm younger doesn't mean I don't know what I want'. They wanted to tell their elders (and all three of us older women could have been their mothers), 'You don't know how it works!' They were resentful that, in our generation, we had been able to go to university and get support to start our professional lives, while these students would be burdened for years with educational debt.

For one older participant this difference was not easy: 'There's some reluctance to, to think about you as being different because you're younger … Maybe it's just my, my reluctance to acknowledge difference … 'cause difference can lead to conflict'. This comment seemed to touch on the underlying dynamic in the group, which had not been spoken about, which was the nature of the extreme conflict between generations.

The second dream drawing was by one of the youngest participants and depicted her in a swimming pool with a shark nearby. Here, perhaps the conflict was more out in the open. An older woman noted: 'You could be out of your depth in certain ways'. And there were very reflective comments by two participants, one younger and one older:

> I really enjoy people that are older than me talking about their experiences, what they've learnt, how they've dealt with situations, because I can really learn from that. But on the other hand, I kind of feel sad because although I can still live it, like that time is over for them …

> I kind of feel sad or guilty that I like can do it now, but that time is gone for them.
>
> I really know what that phrase being 'over the hill' means. I really have that experience inside, you know. The feeling that actually I've reached my zenith and now there is no other way but down, down all the way to the bottom … . which is a scary sort of feeling … . I can't actually go back, you know. It has to carry on to the end of that arc, wherever that may be.

In other words, the older people had the experience and wisdom but less time. And the younger people had all the time in the world, but without the advantages that we had enjoyed. It was a no-win situation.

When reflecting on this experience after the workshop, I noted that I took a particularly motherly role with one of the youngest participants, which was commented on. This was definitely an act of going out of the role, which could be seen as an enactment of the generational issues in the group. By behaving in a motherly way, I was falling into a familiar generational dynamic and creating a private pair, which might have felt comfortable, but went against the task of the work. So I was enacting the very issue of the group, the generational divide.[1]

In fact, it seemed that we as a group all participated in creating a split between the generations. We all colluded in having the participant in the middle (presumably the safest one of us) present the first dream drawing. She served as a mediating figure in that sense, and perhaps it was easier to work first with her dream drawing rather than the one by the younger person. Nevertheless, although the first dream drawer was easily ten years older than the two youngest members, we lumped them all together as the 'young' group. She herself colluded with this, noting in her interview that as a group participant, she was 'feeling myself a lot younger than I was'.

Thus I would say that these extreme tensions between the generations (feelings of motherliness, feelings that the younger participants are not getting a good deal in society, or feeling dismissed by the older generation) were so strong that they dominated the system at the expense of the course. And while before this session, most participants were having difficulty identifying a research question, following the session, almost all were able to.

The potent generational issues were impeding the group's ability to get on with the task. In the workshop, however, these issues could be explored through the dream drawings. Then some of the anxiety was alleviated enough for the participants (including myself) to focus on the assignment for the course.

SDD as a doctoral research method

Neo Pule, a psychology lecturer at the University of the Free State in Bloemfontein, has always been a leader, even as a child. As a student in a predominantly white university, she was the first black person to run for the position of student leader. Although she lost that election, another black student, whom she supported, won the following year.

For her doctoral thesis, she wanted to focus on student leadership in South Africa in order to learn more about the major challenges of taking these roles. Student leadership in South Africa is important for at least two major reasons. First, it is an avenue for work experience, so it spells future opportunity. Second, as she puts it, 'It is a role that allows students to take the bull by the horns ... the bull is the injustice of the South African history'.

The Department of Higher Education has a policy that student leaders are to be involved in every decision a university makes, which makes student leadership a role of influence and status. However, even with this mandate, Pule says they are still 'small beings in a big system', interacting directly with major authority figures, such as professors and principals. Although they are officially 'on the same eye level' with them, many find it quite difficult to take this role successfully.

In preparing for her doctoral work, Pule found traditional research methods such as questionnaires and interviews inadequate for getting to the deeper experience of student leadership. So she decided to use SDD as her research method.

Her students responded well to the method. Using it, they were able to speak freely about contentious issues – and student leadership in South Africa is contentious. She found that through working with SDD, student leaders became quite aware of the charged feelings and special difficulties of taking this role. And she says it has helped make 'what is difficult to articulate tangible. Students were all of a sudden speaking about things that they fantasize about or that is unspoken or roaming around in their unconscious, through the dream drawings'.

This method has especially helped them to recognise and acknowledge 'the unpopular things to articulate about SA history, where they find themselves. Post the promises that came with the rainbow nation'.

In Figure 10.3, the dream drawing by one of her students shows none of the rainbow colours. It expresses the sense of possible birth (pregnant figure) surrounded by a dark set of lines, possibly representing the difficult past.[2]

As Pule is a lecturer and is running these groups in a university environment, she has adapted the reflection process to a more familiar way of working in university classrooms. After each drawing is worked on, she records on a whiteboard the reflections and thoughts of the group in answer to the question: 'What can we say about student leadership?'

At the end of the workshop, after all drawings have been worked with, she integrates the day's work by asking them to look at all the comments on the whiteboard and to bring out the main points. She strives to leave them with tangibles, 'things to walk away with'. Thus she asks them: 'What can we do further? What steps can we take? What questions can we explore? What further thoughts do we need to develop?'

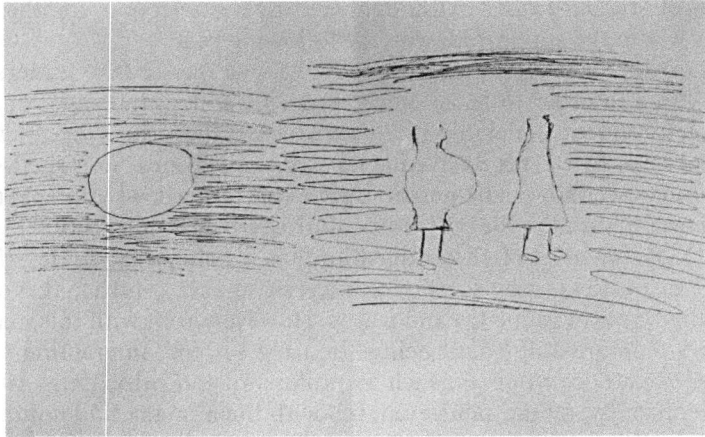

Figure 10.3 Pregnant

In using the whiteboard, the experience feels more familiar to them and students do not leave these intense workshops without intent and purpose. As Pule puts it: 'I take SDD as a consulting tool. Leave them with something to touch. Something I can know, be aware of, I can take further on my own'.

Using SDD for my own learning

I thought I would end this book by describing my own personal experience of SDD.

Here in my home city of Solingen, I have three friends who are all transitioning into retirement. I offered them the chance to use their dreams and their drawings to support them through this major life transition.

Of course, I expected to take the role of facilitator and did so for our first session. However, just before our second session, which was held about six weeks later, I had a dream that I realised was very important.

When we met for the second time, I told the group that I also had a dream drawing (Figure 10.4), and they encouraged me to share it. I asked one of the group members to facilitate.

I then described how, in this dream, I am in the role of lecturer, facing a group of students who are sitting in rows of seats that slope upwards, as in a traditional lecture hall. There is a set of steps in the middle, and the students sit in two groups. Most of the seats are filled. As I look up, there is a group of students who are badly misbehaving, and the local security people have come in to remove them.

I observe this commotion.

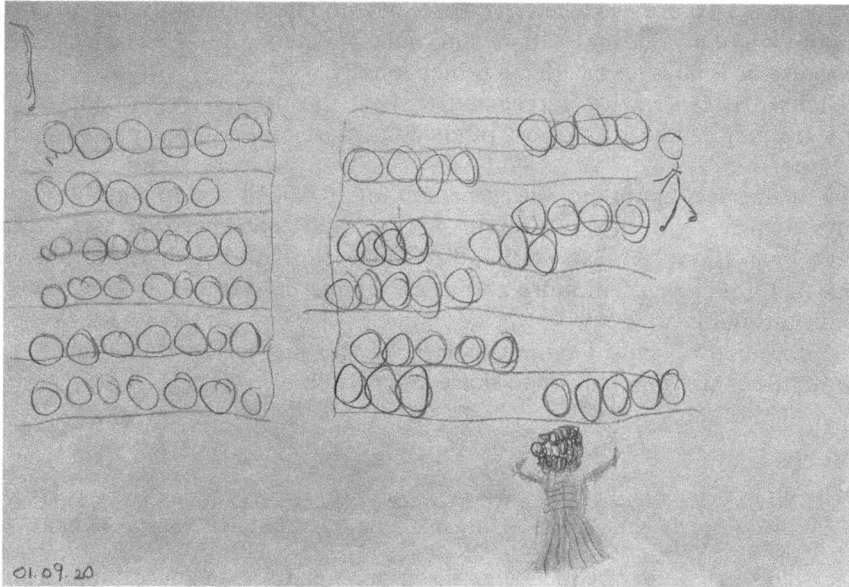

Figure 10.4 Frozen in fear

I then become terrified that I must teach this group of students, and I haven't prepared anything in advance. I don't have anything to offer. There is nothing inside of me to offer. I am frozen in fear.

My back is against a wall and I can't get out.

The associations and responses of the group made me realise what this dream was telling me. For over two decades, my husband and I had worked together as partners. Together we formed a great professional team and offered consultation and workshops all over the world. All these workshops had in common the idea of accessing the unconscious processes in groups through creative means, such as drawings (Organisational Role Analysis), photographs (Social Photo-Matrix) and dreams (SDD and Social Dreaming). The work was always very creative and satisfying.

However, my husband was stricken with early dementia a few years ago, and we have not been able to work together since then.

When we worked together, we had developed a kind of co-partnering system. My husband was the content man, providing the theory and the intellectual material. In contrast, I was always focused on the process. I would design our workshops and could work very well with people in a group situation. I was the process person; he was the content person.

Although I had always (and still do) teach university courses by myself, what this dream drawing reveals is the terrible sadness and fear and emptiness I experience when not working with my husband. In this dream, I cannot find my internal self, my internal competency. I feel I have lost it all because he is no longer with me professionally.

This dream drawing forced me to face the deeply tragic aspects of my transition: the loss of an intellectual and professional partner and partnership.

I found this experience very profound. It helped me to finally allow myself to recognise this enormous loss (not just on a personal basis, but on a professional one as well) and to move on. And I really have moved on, as I am engaged in more and more interesting projects (on my own!) internationally.

I can only say that having experienced this method myself, I feel very grateful for the opportunity to share it in this book.

Notes

1 Mersky, R. (2001) 'Falling from Grace' – When consultants go out of role: enactment in the service of organizational consultancy. *Socio-Analysis*. 3, pp. 37–53.
2 This photo appeared in Pule's dissertation and was obtained through the University of South Africa.

Bibliography

Armstrong, D. (1996) The recovery of meaning. Paper presented to the annual symposium of the International Society for the Psychoanalytic Study of Organizations, 'Organisation 2000: Psychoanalytic Perspectives', June 1996, New York.

Arnheim, R. (1969) *Visual Thinking*. Berkeley: University of California Press.

Benjamin, J. (2004) Beyond doer and done to: An intersubjective view of thirdness. *Psychoanalytic Quarterly*. 73, pp. 5–46.

Bion, W.R. (1961) *Experiences in Groups and Other Papers*. London: Tavistock Publications.

Bion, W.R. (1991) *Learning from Experience*. Northvale, NJ: Jason Aronson. (Original work published 1962).

Bollas, C. (2007) *The Freudian Moment: Second Edition*. Reprint. London: Karnac, 2013.

Bollas, C. (2011) *The Christopher Bollas Reader*. London: Routledge.

Brakel, L.A. (1993) Shall drawing become part of free association? – Proposal for a modification in psychoanalytic technique. *Journal of the American Psychoanalytic Association*. 41, pp. 359–393.

Cardona, F. (2020) *Work Matters: Consulting to Leaders and Organizations in the Tavistock Tradition*. London: Routledge.

Coxhead, D. and Hiller, S. (1976) *Dreams: Visions of the Night*. New York: Thames and Hudson.

Eames, A. (2012) Embedded drawing. In: Garner, S., ed., *Writing on Drawing: Essays on Drawing Practice and Research*. Bristol: Intellect, pp. 125–139.

Edgar, I.R. (1999) The imagework method in health and social science research. *Qualitative Health Research*. 9, pp. 198–211.

Fay, B. (2013) *What Is Drawing – A Continuous Incompleteness*. Dublin: Irish Museum of Modern Art.

Fischer, C. (1957) A study of the preliminary stages of the constructions of dreams and images. *Journal of the American Psychoanalytic Association*. 5, pp. 5–60.

French, R. (1997) The teacher as container of anxiety: Psychoanalysis and the role of teacher. *Journal of Management Education*. 21 (4), pp. 483–495.

Freud, S. (1900) *The Interpretation of Dreams*. S.E. Volume 4–5. Reprint. Middlesex: Penguin, 1976.

Furth, G.M. (1988) *The Secret World of Drawings – Healing Through Art*. Boston: Sigo Press.

Gilmore, S. and Warren, S. (2007) Emotion online: Experience of teaching in a virtual learning environment. *Human Relations.* 60 (4), pp. 581–608.

Gosling, J. and Case, P. (2013) Social dreaming and ecocentric ethics: Sources of non-rational insight in the face of climate change catastrophe. *Organization.* 20 (5), pp. 705–721.

Grisoni, L. (2012) Poem houses: An arts based inquiry into making a transitional artefact to explore shifting understandings and new insights in presentational knowing. *Journal of Organizational Aesthetics* 1 (1), pp. 11–25.

Haartman, K. (no date) *Review of Grotstein, James S. (2000). Who Is the Dreamer Who Dreams the Dream?* Hillsdale: The Analytic Press. *Kleinian Studies Ejournal.* http://www.psychoanalysis-and-therapy.com/human_nature/ksej/hartmangrotstein.html. [accessed 08.09.2014].

Hau, S. (2004) *Träume zeichnen: Über die visuelle Darstellung von Traumbildern.* Tübingen: edition discord.

Hoss, R. (2019a) Private email correspondence.

Hoss, R. (2019b) *Dream Language: A Handbook for Dreamwork* (2nd ed.). (PDF version.)

Jung, C.G. (1930) *The Red Book: Liber Novus.* Reprint. New York: The Philemon Foundation & W.W. Norton & Co, 2009.

Jung, C.G. (1961) *Memories, Dreams, Reflections.* Reprint. London: Fontana, 1995.

Langer, S. (1960) *Philosophy in a New Key.* Cambridge: Harvard University Press.

Lawrence, W.G. (2003) Social dreaming as sustained thinking. *Human Relations.* 56 (5), pp. 609–624.

Long, S. (2013) *Socioanalytic Methods: Discovering the Hidden in Organisations and Social Systems* (1st ed.). Routledge. https://doi.org/10.4324/9780429480355

Mersky, R. (2001) 'Falling from Grace' – When consultants go out of role: Enactment in the service of organizational consultancy. *Socio-Analysis.* 3, pp. 37–53.

Mersky, R. (2006) Organizational role analysis by telephone: The client I met only once. In: Newton, J., Long, S. and Sievers, B., eds., *Coaching in Depth: The Organizational Role Analysis Approach.* London: Karnac, pp. 113–125.

Morgan-Jones, R.J. (2022 forthcoming) The Trilogy Matrix event: A setting for integrating the study of large social system dynamics from different dimensions. In: Hopper, E. and Weinberg, H., eds., *The Social Unconscious in Persons, Groups and Societies: Clinical Implications – Volume 4.* London: Routledge.

Newton, J. (1999) Clinging to the MBA syndicate: Shallowness and 'Second Skin' learning in management education. *Socio-Analysis.* 1 (2), pp. 151–155.

Perls, F. (1970) Dream seminars. In: Fagan, J. and Shepherd, I.L., eds., *Gestalt Therapy Now.* New York: Harper & Row, pp. 204–233.

Pines, M. (1994) The group-as-a-whole. In: Brown, D. and Zinken, L., eds., *Developments in Group-Analytic Theory.* London: Routledge, pp. 47–59.

Rosenberg, T. (2012) New beginnings and monstrous births: Notes toward an appreciation of ideational drawing. In: Garner, S., ed., *Writing on Drawing: Essays on Drawing Practice and Research.* Bristol: Intellect, pp. 109–124.

Sapochnik, C. (2012) The use of drawing as a research tool in social research [lecture to UWE post graduate psycho-social group seminar]. University of West England, Bristol, UK. 14 November.

Sapochnik, C. (2013) Drawing below the surface: eliciting tacit knowledge in social science research. *Tracey.* Special Edition Edition developed from selected papers at the 2012 Doctoral Research Conference (DRC) at Loughborough University, pp. 1–22.

Schredl, M. (2019) Typical dream themes. In: Hoss, R, Valli, K. and Gongloff, R., eds., *Dreams: Understanding Biology, Psychology, and Culture. Volume 1*. Santa Barbara: ABC-CLIO, pp. 180–187.

Shafton, A. (1995) *Dream Reader: Contemporary Approaches to the Understanding of Dreams*. Albany, NY: SUNY Press.

Sievers, B. (2013) Thinking organizations through photographs: The social photo-matrix as a method for understanding organizations in depth. In: Long, S., ed., *Socioanalytic Methods: Discovering the Hidden in Organisations*. London: Karnac, pp. 129–151.

Solms, M. (2014) *Brain mechanisms underpinning some social processes*. [plenary presentation at annual conference of the Organisation for Promoting Understanding of Society (OPUS)] London, UK. 22 November.

Taylor, A. (2012) Forward – Re: Positioning drawing. In: Garner, S., ed., *Writing on Drawing: Essays on Drawing Practice and Research*. Bristol: Intellect, pp. 9–11.

The Companion Bible. (1974) Grand Rapids: Zondervan Bible Publishers.

Ullman, M. (1960) The social roots of the dream. *The American Journal of Psychoanalysis*. 20, pp. 180–196.

Van Alphen, E. (2012) Looking at drawing: Theoretical distinctions and their usefulness. In: Garner, S., ed., *Writing on Drawing: Essays on Drawing Practice and Research*. Bristol: Intellect, pp. 59–70.

Vince, R. and Broussine, M. (1996) Paradox, defense, attachment – Accessing and working with emotions and relations underlying organizational change. *Organization Studies*. 17, pp. 1–21.

Walde, C. (1999) Dream interpretation in a prosperous age? In: Shulman, D. and Stroumsa, G.G., eds., *Dream Cultures: Explorations in the Comparative History of Dreaming*. New York: Oxford University Press, pp. 121–142.

Walker, M. (2017) *Why We Sleep: The New Science of Sleep and Dreams*. UK: Penguin.

Winnicott, D.W. (1967) The location of cultural experience. *International Journal of Psychoanalysis*. 48, pp. 368–372.

Winnicott, D.W. (1971) *Playing and Reality*. Reprint. London: Routledge, 1996.

Zelizer, B. (2004) The voice of the visual in memory. In: Phillips, K., ed., *Framing Public Memory*. Tuscaloosa: The University of Alabama Press, pp. 157–186.

Index

For Product Safety Concerns and Information please contact our EU
representative GPSR@taylorandfrancis.com
Taylor & Francis Verlag GmbH, Kaufingerstraße 24, 80331 München, Germany